I0129348

Dragon with a Cane

中国龙策杖而行

Profiles in Ageing: China's Forgotten Generation
岁月的轮廓--中国被遗忘的一代

by
Bromme Hampton Cole
柯 博 明

The author's second book in a series describing China's unique demographic journey

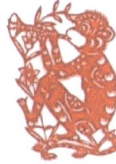

USA Edition 2016

z

Published by: Patient Lao Wei Publications (Shanghai) in cooperation with

HHH Media Ltd., Hong Kong

LCCN:
ISBN-13: 978-0-9856871-2-0

This book is dedicated to my three children.
I wake up each day thinking of you and those
many special moments we have shared:

Mackenzie Kathryn

The many gymnastics events we traveled to together especially the time
when we had to find a doctor to relieve your eye pain just in time
for you to perform then win your match!

Bromme Hampton II

All the chess matches we attended together, our mind-melds and especially
the time when you won first place in New York City!

Waverly Hayes

Those many evenings in Amagansett on the beach, cooking S'mores around
the fire pit and I saved you as you slipped and nearly fell in...

I love you each with every fiber of my being.

"Do not go gentle into that good night,
Old age should burn and rave at close of day;
Rage, rage against the dying of the light"

Dylan Thomas

"A man is a God in ruins. When men are innocent,
life shall be longer, and shall pass into the immortal,
as gently as we awake from dreams."

Ralph Waldo Emerson

Other publications by the Author:

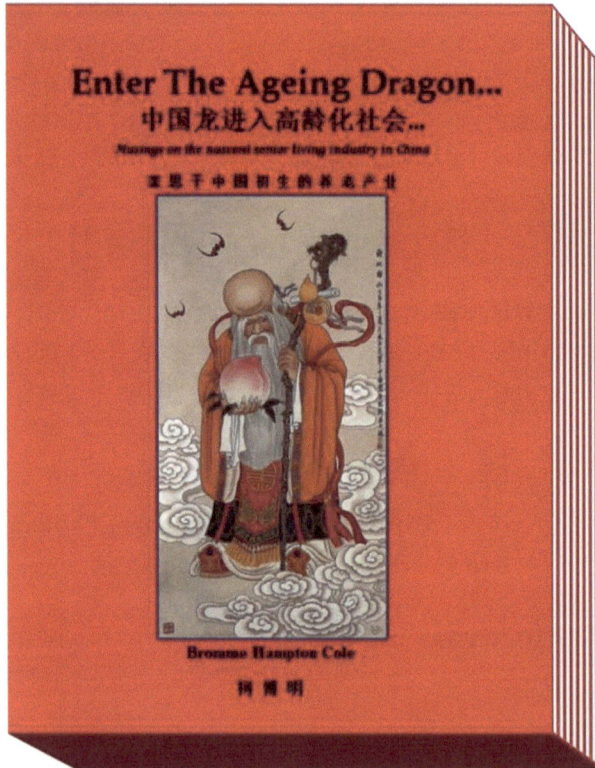

Published 2013

Available on Amazon.com

To be released in 2018

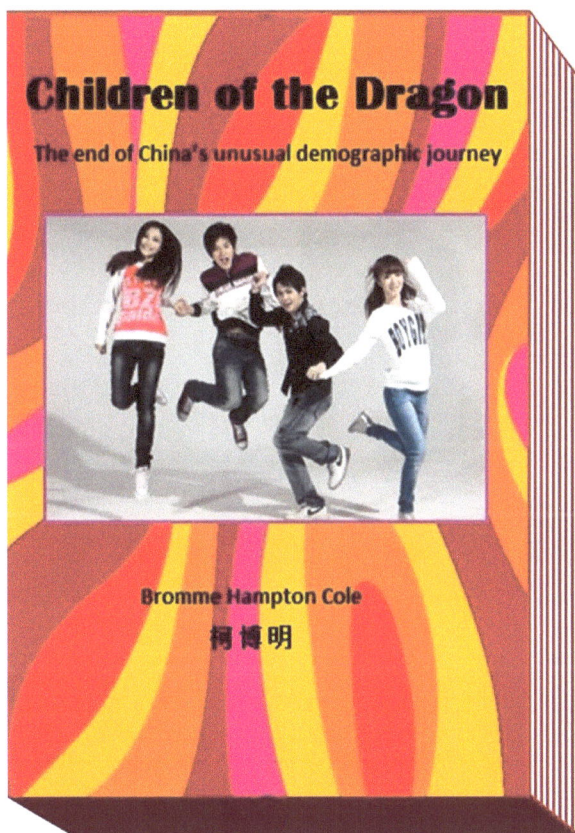

Essential Contributors

English Edition Editors:
Stewart Cole
Nancy Cole
Jack Cumming

Chinese Edition Translators:
Jasmine Si (6, introduction and theory)
Sherry Xu (2)

Chinese Edition Editors:
Zhang Jian
Jessica Yang

Chinese Titles:
Jasmine Sun
Liao Shi Ying
Zhang Jian

Artwork:
Gustavo Glusman
Wang Yaoyi
Bruce Zhang
Raymond Li

Constructive Criticism:
Anna Birthe Bach
Jeremy Nixey
Susie Bates
Snezhana Chernova
Heather Thompson
Allison Bourke

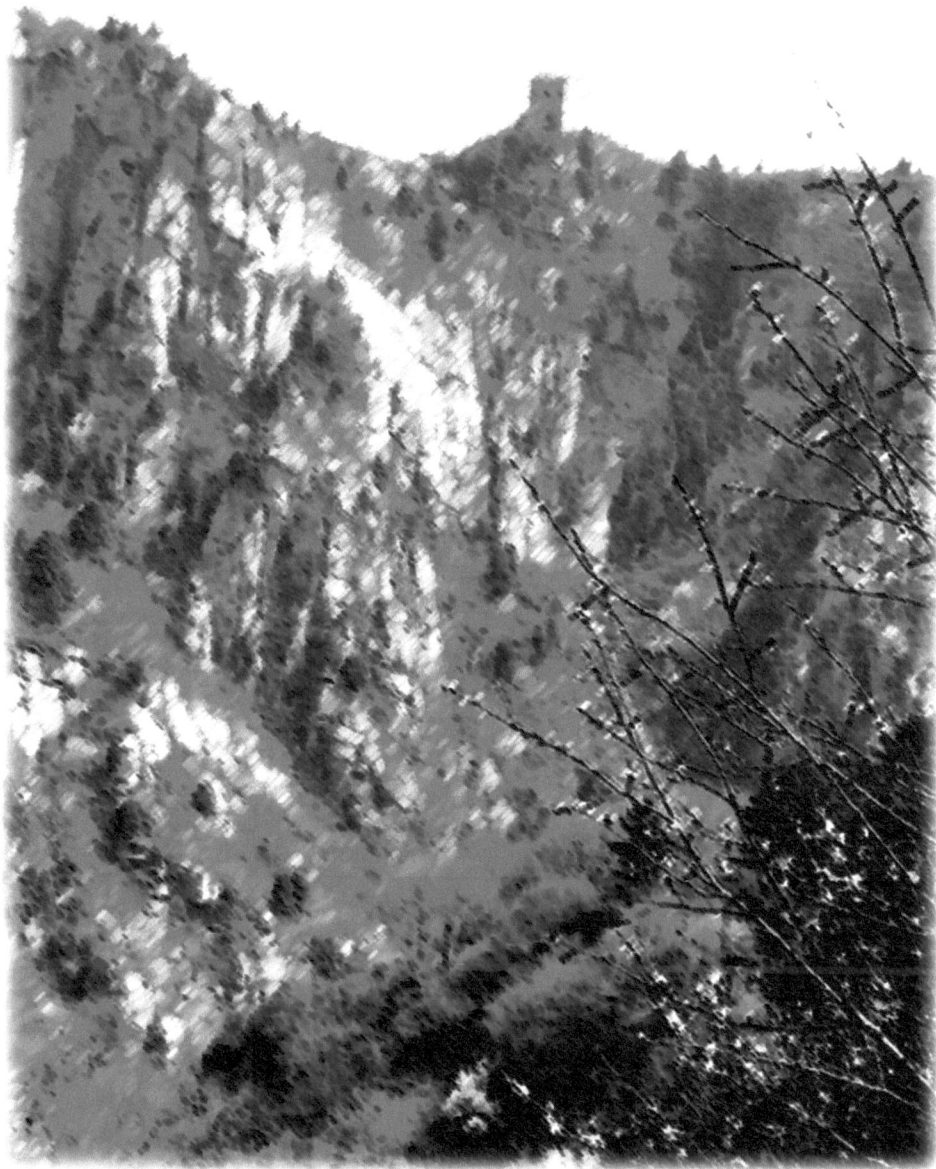

This book is inscribed to:

Special thanks to the following friends. Each of you played a different yet equally important role in the realization of this book.

First, to all my Profiles; the men and women I interviewed. Your inspirational stories stimulated me to no end – Thank you.

Second, to my printer and publisher.

Third, to my Staff - Cherry Chen, Callum Xia, Gavin Guo, Cassie Huang, TT Wang,

Fourth, to my friends whose encouragement and support was critical to this book's realization – Beek and his introduction to Wang Deshun, Ma Ying for all her support, Bob Wang and his comments on Buddhist thought, Lulu Xiong and her introduction to Su Xiu, Brad Perkins and his lovely wife, Phyllis Perkins for all their support and compliments!, Jeremey Nixey for his critical eye, DJ QQ for her contribution…, once again to Elaine Young for the advice she gave me over 6 years ago, Joseph Christian for his thoughts and ideas on an early manuscript, David and Jared from La Bota: good wine and great times, The Grammarian: Susie Q. Bates!, Caron Sprake for her support from afar, Natty Sanz for her encouragement, Antonella Tesei per il tuo sostegno!, Steven Bielinski for his comments on Lavender Dynasty, my translators: Jasmine Si (6 stories) and Sherry Xu (2 stories), Li Guohong for her encouragement and agreement that my theory holds promise, Jacob Juul Hansen, Hanna Liv Leanderdal, Mr. Zhang from Yichang, Sofia Shakil from ADB and all her support, Eloisa "Ave" Avila from Waterman, Bill Zhang from UBM, my good friend: Anna Birthe Bach, Fara Gold who always is complimentary and so sincere about it, Sheena for her encouragement, Michael Qu for his thoughts on my endeavor, Zhang Yu at CDIA, Allison Bourke for her helpful comments, Jane Zhang for her edits and inspiration for the theory, Jose Vilchez for his hard work, Marc Wortmann for his conversations on dementia, Matthew Mommer, Lisa Jiang for inspiration, Katie Sloan and Zhang Naizi for their Prefaces, Dr. Ramon Murphy, Zhou Yupeng, former mayor of Shanghai, Catherine Hua from Jinling Tianquan Lake, and my good friend Kevin Ryan, and to my wife Tricia for her inexhaustible perseverance.

Table of Contents

Chinese Preface

This book is a collection of stories describing the spiritual aspect of elderly people's life in China. Each case has illuminated an old person's persistence in the pursuance of his or her ideal with a reflection back in his or her own life. Their personal profiles presented in these stories provide us, as aged-care professionals, with more insights into the senior's spiritual world and cultural life together with their perceptions of the universe. In other words, we are able to understand more about each elderly individual's life journey that is, certainly, associated with politics, culture, and social transformations across different era through which they lived their long life. Indeed, readers will be very much touched by their values, life courage, self-reliance, independent will, self-respect, dignity, joy and love.

As a senior executive with over 20 years' experience in the elderly care service industry, as a doctor and socio-psychologist, I strongly feel the publication of this book will have profound impact for China aged-care industry professionals. After reading this book, care managers would at least appreciate two principals: in order to offer better services for seniors, it is vital to essentially show true respect to those elders' life style and personal expression and to pay attention to their opinions on the society and their understanding of the world. For the front-line care workers, this book will help them grasp the diverse and dynamic care needs of elderly people. By doing so, this will also facilitate a better match of supply and demand in terms of an approximate, quality, humanitarian approach towards elderly care services.

For general readers, from the stories in this book they will acquire a large amount of information about what the elders think and the hopes the elder generation place on the younger generation. With a clear picture of these thoughts and expectations, the young people will have a good reference point to provide seniors with due care and respect: in all continuance of filial piety. We sincerely acknowledge and appreciate that all human beings have a responsibility for caring and devoting their hearts for the old people. We wish the elders a healthy body and mind as well as a joyful life with happiness and dignity. With the love from across the generations, from children to mature care workers, the sunset will surely continue to be shining with beauty and pleasure.

Dr. Zhang Naizi – Dean Emeritus 3rd Social Welfare Institute of Shanghai

English Preface

This collection of stories is poignant and revealing. It offers a unique window into the lives of those who are aging in China today. The forces of change in China - culturally, economically, politically - over the past decade are evident in the particular circumstances of the individuals about whom Bromme Hampton Cole has written. Each is different one from the other, but all are connected by the mere fact that they have lived long and eventful lives. The influence of Chinese culture is pronounced, but we know that the process of ageing is a universal experience. Those in other countries will bring a different set of experiences with them as they age but, fundamentally, aging is a stage of life. As with other stages of life, aging is full of opportunity, challenges, joys and sorrows. These stories reinforce all this about aging and more.

Katie Smith Sloan

President and CEO, LeadingAge

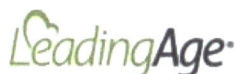

*Leading**Age**·*

LIFE by Wang Yaoyi

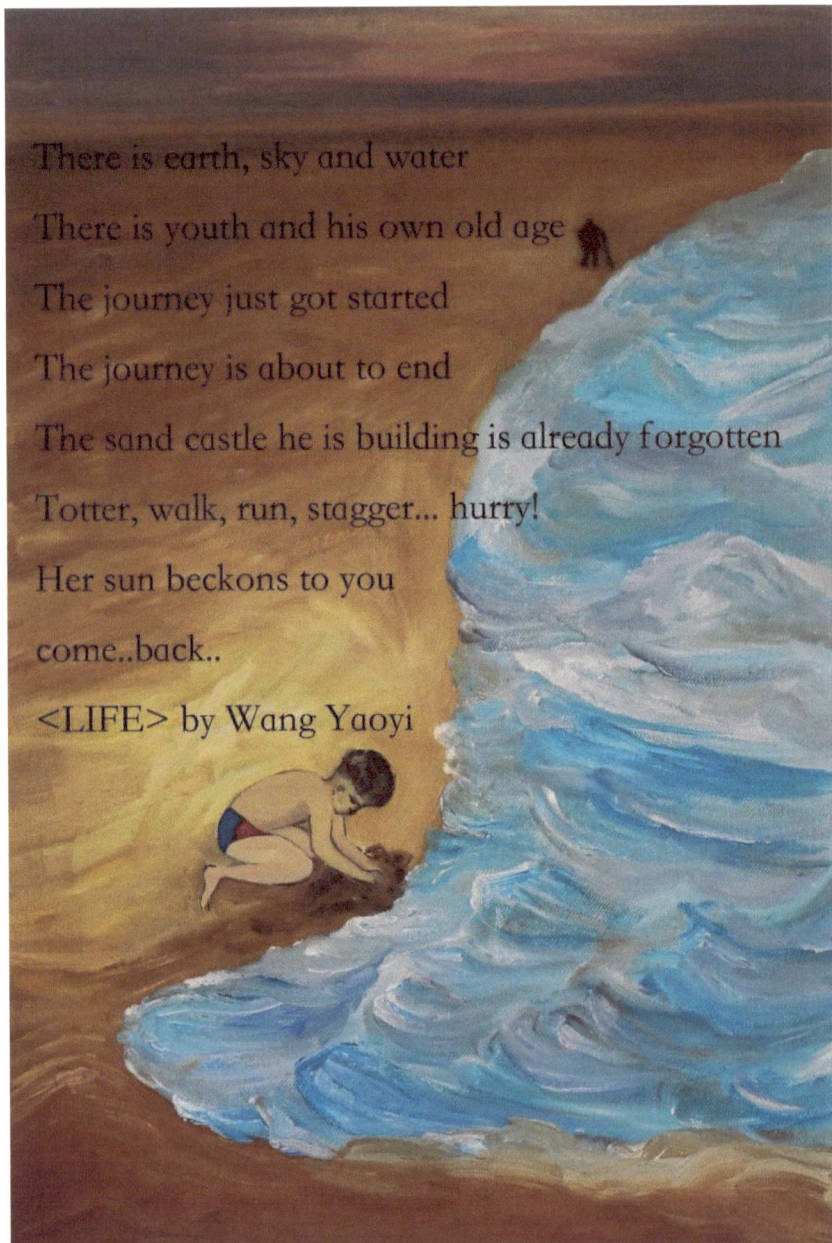

There is earth, sky and water

There is youth and his own old age

The journey just got started

The journey is about to end

The sand castle he is building is already forgotten

Totter, walk, run, stagger... hurry!

Her sun beckons to you

come..back..

<LIFE> by Wang Yaoyi

Author's Preface

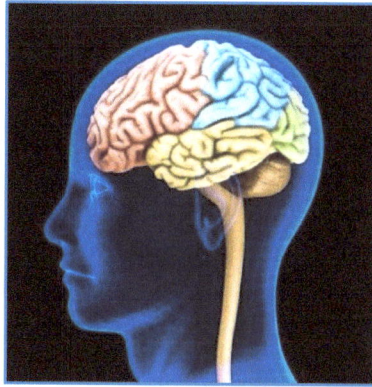

On the back cover, I call this book an ethnographic manifesto.

(I'll let that sink in for a minute...)

Here's why: Ahead of you are eight stories all based on interviews I conducted of elderly Chinese men and women[1]. They are true accounts of my discussions along with understandable edits for style, improved environment and of course, enriched for poignancy of metaphor. The profiles are close accountings of the subject's lives with a focus on the challenges they face today as they age. All my interviewees were born around the founding of the CPC and most are or were over the age of 75 when I sat with them. Some have died since I completed their interviews. But in all, their lives have spanned an extraordinary period of Chinese modern history in terms of cultural, political and societal development; hence my claim of ethnography. Regarding the manifesto attribute, this book is a public declaration that sums the weight of my interviewee's

---

[1] I did not interview Zhu Xiuyu, Wang Xiaohong or Shen Dihan. I produced their stories from third party discussions.

experiences as older Chinese. Everyone in China is talking about senior care today but the personal journeys of the elderly, their vulnerabilities as humans, their relationships, their hopes and fears, without the labels of frailty or incompetency, are largely ignored. No one is discussing these issues; so this book is their voice, their petition...their moment of advocacy and thus a manifesto on their behalf.

In the next chapter I will introduce an idea that came about at the end of my interviews and their final written recording. The concept, which is actually a theory, changes the tone of the book and introduces an alternative use for all the profiles. I will leave it up to you the reader, which story line you prefer: the profiles as records of the elderly Chinese experience in the early 21st Century, or the interviews as case studies supporting a theory on Chinese ageing, or perhaps both...as a doubly stimulating piece of literature.

A mighty French philosopher once said, as only as this breed of people can proclaim, "Demography is Destiny". I like this quote...it has the ring of authenticity. It is a big, existential statement to be sure but it also has a genuineness that is undeniable. I don't know if China's demography will determine its future and that isn't what this book is about nor was it my objective when I set about writing. My purpose here is much simpler: first, I enjoy writing about things for which I care; second, this is a story that needed to be told: the elderly Chinese, after a century of sacrifice, deserve their voices to be heard; and third, I wanted to write a book that offered a near opposite perspective of the industry compared with my first book yet keep it relevant to aged care. Shortly after the publication of "_Enter the Ageing Dragon_" people often asked me if I were planning on a Part Two. Frankly, I found the notion of writing a sequel to be confining, as if I had been trapped by the success of my first book and unable to create something wholly different. Reader press on: *"Dragon with a Cane"* is uniquely different. So, collectively, these were my motivations.

In sum, I want to say that this is not a judgmental or disparaging analysis of anything in China. In fact, I have enormous admiration for what China is doing to address care for their elderly; I am certain they will find a successful path on their journey and I am hopeful, my efforts here have helped in some small way.

Enjoy the book.

Bromme Hampton Cole
柯 博 明
August 18, 2016

9 Essential Relationships for Ageing

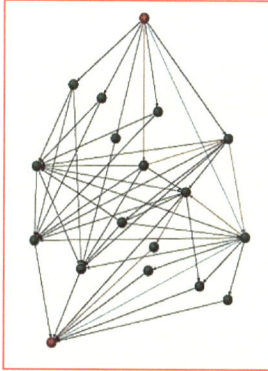

I began to write this book in mid-2014. As I finished each interview and assembled my notes into distinct chapters, trends and similarities emerged among from my interviewee's voices. Points of commonality appeared as they spoke about their experiences and relationships. What had begun merely as an exploration into the intimate lives of the elderly materialized into a set of observable facts and describable phenomena; all of which served as fundamental building blocks to articulate something we all recognize as important. So, as you begin to read, consider the profiles as case studies also as they present a considerable data set. The information the case studies have revealed has given rise to a competing, parallel narrative: namely a social theory on what modern ageing in China is and the elemental components that constitute growing old successfully. And by successful, I mean happy with as much longevity as is natural. In this regard, the case studies serve as effective research only told in a less clinical manner as one might find in proper research.

My theory suggests that there are fundamental social interactions and relationships that define robust old age. I call it *The Social Engagement*

Theory for Chinese Ageing and it is based on nine basic relationships which are essential to the Chinese elderly experience. The 9 Essential Relationships provide an explanatory framework for my observations on ageing in China and the case studies support and illustrate them; indeed they are my empirical proofs. Over the years while in China, I have witnessed each of these nine relationships among the elderly and seen the benefit of their presence and consequence of their absence. The compilation of the case studies and their analysis was the primary source for my development of the 9 Essential Relationships.

The 9 Essential Relationships, in varying proportions, need to be constants in the lives of the elderly. That's not to suggest that each of the Essential Relationships must be present. If fact, many people can live long lives with just some of them. In the case studies that follow will see just that; how some have compensated for the lack of many Essential Relationships and continue to live in a state of equilibrium. But it isn't necessarily the lack or presence of Essential Relationships that matters most. It is the transition of an Essential Relationship, the loss (Negative Transition) or acquisition (Positive Transition) which is profound. The failure of an Essential Relationship produces chaos, it is emotionally disruptive and, depending on the how many Essential Relationships remain in that person's life, it can be terminal. On the other hand however, the acquisition of an Essential Relationship is an interesting phenomenon; it may lengthen life, with certainty it adds joy and richness to an elderly person's experience. It is rare, but it happens: in fact my interviews demonstrate this in four instances. When older people can add an Essential Relationship to their life, it is like the elixir of longevity. Of course, Positive or Negative Transitions are temporary, what is more expected and preferable is a balance. In all, my 9 Essential Relationships are really just the beginning of this concept of a social theory on ageing. I am certain that after this book, there will come revised, much improved considerations, all more scientific, of my hypothesis and I welcome it.

Below, I have defined the 9 Essential Relationships. In the body of this book, after each case study, I distribute each of them in the context of my perception of the interviewee in tabular format along with a brief explanation for my decision. I allocate the Essential Relationships into three categories: A) <u>Has</u>: This category lists those possessed by the subject at the time of interview, B) <u>Has not</u>: in this list, I set forth the Essential Relationships which the subject lacks, and in between, C) <u>Negative/Positive Transition</u>: this column lists those that are undergoing a conversion between Has and Has Not. The distribution of Essential Relationships into these three categories is based on my understanding of the interviewees alone, it is a subjective analysis as there is really no index, no reference and certainly no laboratory for this evaluation.

9 Essential Relationships

Personal

1) <u>Healthy Mind and Spirituality</u> – Productive use of one's mind each day and an appreciation for one's inner dimension and place in great nature.
2) <u>Healthy Body</u> – Consumption of nourishing food and moderate exercise combined with sufficient health care.
3) <u>Happy Heart and Love</u> – Peace, self-contentment and intimacy.
4) <u>Independence and Courage</u> – Maintain autonomy and self-reliance; the ability or willingness to confront uncertainty.
5) <u>Self-Respect and Dignity</u> – Belief in one's purpose and one's value.
6) <u>Sufficient Wealth</u> – Thrift in all financial matters.

Interpersonal

7) <u>Strong Family Bonds</u> – Foundation of life; all extended family beyond spouse or child.
8) <u>Reliable Friendships</u> – Trustworthy peers with whom to share life's joys and assist with its challenges.
9) <u>Productive Engagement and Community Support</u> – Volunteering and contributions to civic endeavors as well as public reverence of the elderly.

The 9 Essential Relationships can be divided into two sub-categories: Personal Relationships and Interpersonal Relationships. The first six are internal: Healthy Mind and Spirituality, Healthy Body, Happy Heart and Love, Independence and Courage, Self-Respect and Dignity and Sufficient Wealth. These speak to self-knowledge and those things which one has a significant degree of control and influence. The second three are external: Strong Family Bonds, Reliable Friendships and Productive Engagement and Community Support; these are matters which one reaches outward to find. The Interpersonal subset is what we all recognize as our support group. These sub-categories are important when collectively examining the case studies. Findings relevant to the presence of Personal and Interpersonal Relationships and the differences between these sub-categories across all case studies are presented in the Appendix portion of the book. Further, I recognize that the case studies are limited in a number of ways. First there are only eight interviews and conclusions are hard with so small a data set. Second, my discussions with the subjects were not perfectly symmetrical; I used no questionnaire. But access to them and their stories might not have been possible had I taken so sterile an approach.

Before I conclude, we may intuitively appreciate these relationships as vital, but articulating them as I have done here is important for at least one purpose. The theory, and its subsequent development by others, has practical implications for the future of the industry here in China from many perspectives. For example, Chinese elderly care policy makers might contemplate the theory and the insights it provides for the development of long term care insurance strategies and funding of health care training programs. Likewise, facility operators and managers might study the theory for early intervention with at-risk patients and establish more patient centered care programs. I can also visualize specialty employment opportunities such as spiritual care professionals, personal relationship managers and activity engagement specialists. These are only a few ideas for the pragmatic uses of the theory.

Social Engagement Theory for Chinese Ageing

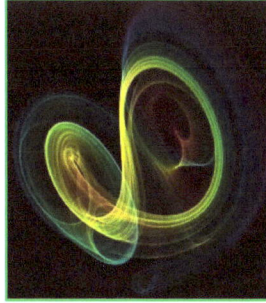

Hypothesis:

As people age, our social interactions become critically important. The elderly develop routines that become the footing of daily life, they depend upon these schedules and they become almost habitual providing internal and external structure to their lives. During these routines, the elderly engage in and practice social relationships, these relationships or engagements are an essential psychological construct that provides security against the fear of social disengagement and ultimately death. The negative or positive transition of these relationships can be traumatic or fulfilling. These relationships are as elemental to the survival of the elderly as are clinical considerations such as morbidity or disease management; indeed the loss of social connections for the elderly could be considered a type of pathology. There are nine of these fundamental social connections which are called the "9 Essential Relationships for Ageing" and are the underpinning of this theory.

> *Corollary 1 - Elderly people can subsist on as few as 3 Essential Relationships.*

Corollary 2 – *The Negative Transition of 2 or more Essential Relationships is difficult to endure.*

Corollary 3 - *The Positive Transition of one or more Essential Relationships is life extending.*

Corollary 4 – *An abundance of Essential Relationships (6 or more) offers a greater social platform to endure the loss of Essential Relationships.*

Corollary 5 – *Clinical intervention or adaptive behavior may compensate for the Negative Transition of an Essential Relationship.*

The Profiles

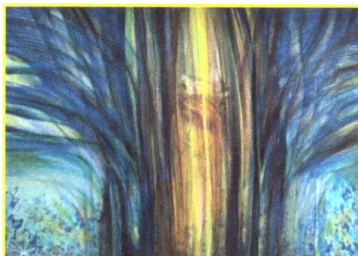

Zhu Xiuyu

A lonely old woman, lost to this world and for reasons that shouldn't be.

Jun and Shishang

A loving couple, dedicated to each other forever, whose end is as tragic as one can imagine.

Wang Xiaohong

The sweetest woman and a victim of circumstances far beyond her control, pays an unfair price.

Mrs. Jiang and her daughter

The inspiring dedication of a daughter to her mother: filial piety in action.

Su Xiu

Everlasting love between husband and wife is rejuvenated after a spouse's death.

Wang Deshun

A lesson in courage from the youngest, old man alive...

Jiabei and Haoming

Two elderly Chinese seniors take a risk and find love.

Shen Dihan

An old man living on borrowed time finds mercy among old friends.

Xiuyu's Epitaph

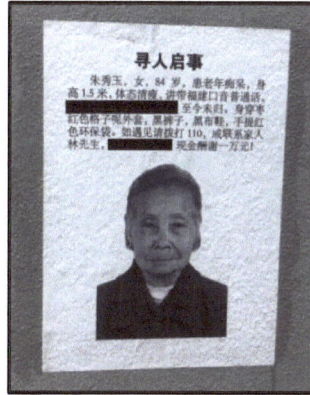

Dementia in China is a real challenge and a challenge at every level imaginable. From the popular Chinese word used to describe the disease to social stigma, lack of preventative care and on to inadequate treatment available to the average person. I have seen a lot of those who suffer from the many kinds of dementia, and like other countries the skill level of care givers varies greatly. But China's biggest difficulty in my opinion is not really their competence or understanding but access to care. The vast majority of those with some sort of dementia have little recourse to the treatment they require. There is no reliable figure of those who suffer in China but if one extrapolates the afflicted population using Western rates of incidence for dementia, today's number must be around 18 million. As China's elderly population expands, that figure will likely grow to over 40 million, or about the population of South Korea.

Meet Zhu Xiuyu whom I know only from this photo. It is a report of a missing person, which I found taped to a public wall used frequently for community notices. Xiuyu, as I will call her, is 84 years old and for three years spent most of her day sitting on the sidewalk, tethered to a stake hammered into the ground next to her daughter's small restaurant of 2 tables and 8 seats on Jian Guo Lu, located in a bustling southeast Shanghai neighborhood. Xiuyu's exact diagnosis was not known but she had profound memory loss; she recognized no one, was mistrustful and at times, hostile. Sometime between breakfast and lunch on the day she disappeared, Xiuyu, in an act of utter hopelessness, freed herself from the tether, removed her shoes and walked away...quietly, unnoticed and forever.

Her daughter, Xicen, was bereft. Immediately after her Xiuyu's disappearance, she closed her restaurant and for two weeks hiked all over Shanghai, frantically searching for her mother. Her feet are still bruised and blistered and bear witness to her hunt. Breathless with desperation...she cried out her mother's name at every corner, choking back her panic, pacing street after street after street. In the past few days, Xicen has given into despair and is resigned to never see her mother again. Her inquiries at the local police produced little more than indifference. She is overwhelmed with grief and crumbles into tears spontaneously, sobbing over her cold stove, holding a picture of her mother to her heaving chest. Speaking with her is hard; anguish has torn her soul apart.

Xicen is 45 and Xiuyu's only daughter. In turn, she was her mother's only care giver and source of support. She works on average a 15 hour day, 7 days a week to eek a meager living from her small stove. If she does not cook, she will perish. There is no male presence in this household: Xiuyu's husband died decades ago and her daughter never married. Xicen, as a single, middle aged woman, is known in Chinese society as one of the millions of "left-over women". She and her mother are poor and the last in line to benefit from the Chinese economic miracle.

Years ago when Xiuyu's disorientation began, Xicen took her to the hospital seeking an appointment; four months later she saw a Doctor. The results were inconclusive. The Doctor was unsure and hesitant to recommend the common treatment of powerful sedatives. Besides, there was no available bed at the local hospital for the resources Xicen had to offer. Unfortunately as simple cook, she lacked sufficient guanxi to call upon others who might be in a position to enable the favor of hastened admission. Yet from Xicen's perspective, Xiuyu's weakening memory was stark and required urgent care. Over the next 3 years, Xiuyu dissolved rapidly. Xicen attempted other visits to the hospital and was repeatedly told that the waiting list was long for beds in the ward that kept old people with "lao nian chi dai", the common term for dementia which translates harshly into "old people's idiotic behavior". It also offers the added cruel nuance of the word "nian" which can mean monster in Mandarin.

In an effort to understand the realities here in China, in a very local sense, of those who suffer from dementia and how their families cope, I spoke with Xicen at length. Much of what she said was not surprising, however the outcome was terrifying. I sat with Xicen for a few hours as she described her mother's decline in visibly traumatic terms. She lurched back and forth as if in a trance. While speaking, Xicen reached out with her left arm; her hand opened and shut, grasping nothing but air as if she were stretching to save her mother from the pull of a monstrous tide. Xicen detailed the separation painfully as her mother drifted further and further towards liminal recognition. Ultimately, Xicen recalled the point of no return... she sat up abruptly, her face white with shock and eyes in an empty stare, she declared..., "Then on that day, she did not recognize me anymore. I was no longer her daughter and she was not my mother. She was simply gone." Xicen lowers her head, she has no more tears only remorse and emptiness; she sat there silent and alone.

Xicen is mystified at her horrifying misfortune. Her mother's disease was painful enough, indeed for both, but now Xiuyu has vanished into a city of 22 million and likely has met her end or soon will. It is a virtual certainty Xicen will never know her mother's fate. Though no official records exist, hundreds of old people go missing each month, a few are found and those within a day or two at most. But after three weeks the chances are nil of recovery much less reunion. Many expire from dehydration, some are victims to hit and run car accidents, a few throw themselves into the foul Huangpu River and others fall prey to more unspeakable crimes. This tragic drama no doubt plays itself out in many different ways all across our ageing world, some places more horrific than others, no doubt. But as the rising tide of China's economic miracle has lifted many boats, one would hope that those who suffer from dementia will not be left to drift away at risk but instead, provided some safe harbor anchorage.

I thanked Xicen for her time, wished her the best and walked out into a cool Shanghai afternoon. To one side of the restaurant lay Xiuyu's tether twisted about a crude iron stake driven into the ground. Its flat, round top is sharp from being pounded into the ground with a massive hammer; its wide diameter prevented the tether from being pulled off. I bend over and examine the rope. I can see frayed ends…and deduce that Xiuyu used the top of the stake to slice through the rope. I then realized she was desperate to escape. I stood up and stepped back to take in the whole scene before I left. On the ground near the stake, scattered about in a trivial way, are Xiuyu's last earthy possessions: a pair of old shoes, a plastic feed bowl and an umbrella to protect her from the sun. To Western sensitivities this is inhumane, but in the context of Xicen's reality and the health care support system available to her, I understand why this happened. There is no blame assign…no one to impugn, it is a tragedy recognized by all involved. It is one whose causes are undergoing an evolution, a massive societal change whose large gears grind away with exasperating slowness, unmindful of damaged cogs like Xiuyu, the only objective being progress. Xiuyu isn't the first to be caught up in these gears nor will she be the last.

The sight is unbearably pathetic; I walk to the end of the street where I purchase a cardboard box. I return to the stake and collect Xiuyu's meager belongings. I brush the dust off her shoes, shake the umbrella and wipe out the bowl as best I can. I then arrange them carefully in the box and reflect on Xiuyu as I close the lid: She was a woman who was no stranger to chaos, born into the unceasing madness of mid-century China. She lived a life full of severe transformation. The cynical reward for her innocence was to be her daughter's unwilling prisoner, robbed of her sanity and ultimately dying a cruel death. Xiuyu never knew peace and was exhausted with this world. I suspect she had a fleeting moment of agonizing clarity, then, in full possession of her destiny she severed the rope knowing it would free her from this life. I stay for a moment, standing next to the contorted rope meditating the end of Xiuyu's story. With the exception of Xicen's memory of her mother, Xiuyu became as though she had never been born and perished as though she had never lived.

I recite Psalm 23[2] solemnly thinking my box is the only burial Xiuyu will have. Leaving it at the doorstep of Xicen's restaurant, I silently turn and walk home.

The Chinese version of this story was translated from English by Sherry Xu

---

[2] Psalm23 - is often taken as an allusion to the eternal life and is frequently read during funeral liturgies in the West. It is reputed to have been authored by King David.

Zhu Xiuyu - Allocation of 9 Essential Relationships

Has	Negative Transition →	Has not
Healthy Body	Self-respect and Dignity	Sufficient Wealth
		Productive Engagement and Community Support
		Independence and Courage
		Reliable Friendships
		Happy Heart and Love
		Healthy Mind and Spirituality
		Strong Family Bonds

Discussion:

I never met Zhu Xiuyu in person but I have pieced together her story based on the account I got from her daughter. Based on this understanding of her I have allocated the 9 Relationships according to the above table.

Xiuyu's story is a tragedy. She likely compensated for the Essential Relationships she lacked by being having her daughter close to her. In my discussion with Xicen, it was clear that neither of them had any meaningful financial resources, relatively few friends and no family other than each other. Obviously Xiuyu was not independent and given her dementia, had no ability to be engaged in the community or friendships. However, there is no reason to believe Xiuyu was not fundamentally healthy other than her dementia. In fact, she was capable of severing the tether, so she must have had strength. Therefore I allocate a healthy body to Xiuyu though it is a precarious existence possessing a single Essential Relationship. In fact this is an insufficient basis on which to carry on with life. Because of her dementia, loss of independence and the lack of other priorities, her dignity and self-respect begin to transit and consequently the will to live.

The Lavender Dynasty

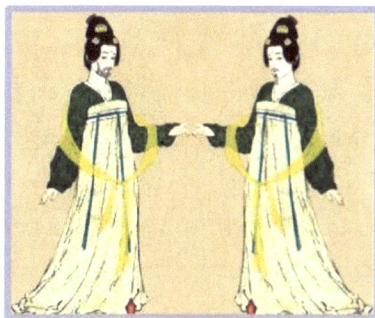

I have a professional colleague who is in the senior living construction business in North America. When I last saw him he told me of his latest project which involved building a senior community for a gay friendly church; the community, of course, would also be gay friendly in fact it would be mostly gay. This wasn't the first I had heard of the emergence of gay senior living, but it was the first time I had spoken to someone who was involved in the realization of such a community. A while ago, the thought struck me that while I know a fair amount about senior care in China, I have no idea how the Chinese gay community is dealing with their health care as they age much less how those who are already infirm and fragile, cope. That is, until now. It took me a while to find a Chinese, elderly gay couple...most of them either have not survived or have been driven so far underground and into obscurity that it is nearly impossible to identify them. This story is the result of my finding such a couple, my interviews with them about their challenges and how they are managing their health in the final stage of their lives. I had three interviews with them but for stylistic purposes I have

condensed them into a single discussion. As it turns out, the
story is far more about their lives than senior care, but there
is good reason for that.

It was the beginning of the end of a long hot Shanghai summer which hadn't seen much rain. And no rain made matters worse. The filth from the roads in Putuo district billowed up behind the growling traffic and, combined with exhaust, was thick enough to asphyxiate. When I arrived at the apartment of Jun and Shishang, it was approaching noon and the sun was high. Their story promised a compelling line and one that I had never encountered before. Jinsong, a friend of mine in Shanghai, put me in touch with Jun and scheduled a series of chats.

I arrived at their apartment building at 430pm on a Tuesday afternoon in late July 2014. My destination was the 17th floor. The building, a type of which there are thousands in Shanghai, was oblong and slab-like, oriented east-west to optimize Feng Shui. The façade had long vertical black water marks from leaking air conditioners which stained the blue pastel panels that stretched from the ground to the top floor. All visual details combined with the heat conspired to render the scene into a tropical urban ghetto.

I stepped into the building's lobby. The walls were scarred by peeling paint, the ash trays next to the elevator overflowed with cigarettes. There were a dozen or so loose newspapers on the floor scattered about. Inside and out, the building looked and felt tired; built with post-Soviet era construction technology to last about 20 years; it was well past its prime.

I pushed the up button on the brass elevator plate and noticed the clear plastic cover was cracked. What plastic was left resembled a half-moon in the way it was cleaved...its long straight edge now worn soft with time, the other piece gone missing years ago, swept up, tossed out and now forgotten. All typical for local apartment buildings in China; small matters and outliers get overlooked in favor of big issues and the majority.

The elevator doors opened and I stepped inside the cab, turned and pressed the 17 button. Thirty-five quiet seconds later the doors opened again and I stepped out into a narrow hall with walls so yellow with age they looked as though one could smell every year they had existed. There was no graffiti just dirt and dust everywhere. I walked to the end of the hallway and found apartment 04, marked in small black numbers. Raising my right hand, I curled my fore finger and knocked. I waited 10 seconds, looked at my watch, and reminded myself I was on time. After another knock and 15 seconds, I could hear a shuffle inside and then the clatter of some apparatus against the floor or walls...then more shuffles...then more clatter. The person behind the door began the process of turning locks. With the metallic clunk of gears, I heard the bottom lock, then the middle lock. The process seemed excessive and felt paranoid to me. Then the door opened a crack and a wizened, old bald man peered out from the narrow opening. He wore a tube around his head that delivered oxygen into his nose.

"Are you Ke?...the young man come to speak to me?", the old man quizzed me, worried about the veracity of my identity.

"Yes, I am Bromme...Jinsong sent me to speak with you", I gave my first name hoping to reassure him that I was indeed the person he was supposed to meet today.

"Come in", he said flatly.

The old man disappeared from the door opening and backed away. As he moved I heard the shuffle and clatter again. I gave the door a small push and it swung wide. I entered the apartment's corridor and closed the door behind me. The old man turned his back turned to me and hobbled down the hallway on a walker. He pushed it a foot or two, then shuffled a step to catch up. As he progressed, the walker banged up against the narrow walls of the hallway and a green oxygen canister swung from a nylon bag strapped to the handlebars.

The old man is Yang Jun. Jun is 76 years old and owns the apartment. He has emphysema and doesn't see well due to the cataracts that fog his vision. Jun is gay and has lived in apartment number 1704 since he and his wife were divorced 20 years ago. He now lives with a man named Shishang and has for 15 years. Though they don't use the word "partners"…that is effectively what they are…instead, they call themselves friends.

Jun maneuvered his walker to his right side and into the living room. He then turned 180 degrees in front of a large recliner seat. With measured precision, he twisted, aimed, leaned back slowly and collapsed into his recliner.

"Please sit down" Jun said, swinging his legs up and adjusting himself in his chair. He directed me to a wooden seat across from where he sat.

"Good afternoon", I tried to smile sensing some annoyance on Jun's part with my presence.

"What do you want to know", Jun was direct…almost surgical.

I wasn't prepared for this question. In fact I was caught off-guard as I had made it clear with Jinsong why I wanted to speak and specifically asked that my purpose be conveyed to Yang Jun.

I began to explain hoping that the answer would come to me, "Well, a few years ago I wrote a book on the senior care industry in China. In that book, I focused on the development of the industry. Today, I am working on another book and I want to explore the challenges of individuals and their stories as they age."

As I uttered these words I became aware of another individual moving about the apartment. In the corner of my left eye, I could see a shadow glide down the hallway quickly. The person was noiseless and I surmised it was Jun's friend, Shishang.

"And what can I tell you that will help in this new endeavor?" Jun pressed me. Again, he had me a bit off guard. He lay there, sinking into his overstuffed recliner...recumbent yet probing.

"Yang Jun...", I began pragmatically, "I know from friends that the plight of gay men in China has been difficult, and although it has improved it remains perilous at times. I want go a step further and understand what the issues are for ageing gay men and their partners." I laid it out for him hoping that it would encourage a meaningful discussion and, of course, learn something that might advance my understanding of ageing in China.

Jun was silent. He stared at me, measuring and thinking. He glanced around the room as if searching for a response from the remnants of his life that were scattered about the table and floor. Old magazines with torn covers, empty pill boxes strewn about the floor, ragged stuffed animals, video cassettes piled up and on a nearby table, sun-bleached, yellowed photos. I compared it to other gay men's apartments I have seen, all fastidiously styled, impeccably clean, bright and carried a *savoire faire* that was immediately identifiable. In frightening contrast, Jun's grim apartment felt like utter defeat.

Then he spoke, "You came to the right place...but I don't think being gay in Shanghai is perilous at all. Being gay, old and sick is...but certainly not just gay."

At first his answer seemed wry and I half expected Jun to smile. But he was deadpan...serious and still. His breathing was labored as he lay there on the plaid recliner. Jun had a curious habit: between breaths he would purse his lips together, wet them with his tongue, squint his eyes and then inhale. When he drew a breath his small chest heaved mightily, he wheezed and fought for every pint of oxygen in the green tank which hung from his walker.

"I thought so" I replied. Continuing, I began to find my ground, "Well, Jun…we have a good deal to speak about…or at least I have a lot to understand. May I begin?"

"Proceed", Jun agreed.

I had a second thought at that moment. As I sat there absorbing the environment, I sensed the situation required that I should not be leading this discussion. Rather, as I looked at Jun, a man who seemed to be shrunken in so many ways, who needed to speak with his own voice and tell his side of life's difficult facts instead of responding to questions that may prejudge the situation. I decided to change direction.

"Jun…", I wondered out loud, "I have an alternative thought. Would you mind if I just sat here and gave you an opportunity to tell me a story about yourself? We are here alone, we don't know one another and I have no judgement to pass here. So…I am hoping…maybe you can find space to here and now to speak as you have never spoken before."

Jun thought for a while. I hoped the silence between us would crystalize into a comfortable place for him.

"Well, not so alone. Shishang is listening to us from the next room so I have to be honest or he won't make dinner for me." Jun smiled for the first time, coughed and narrowed his eyes preparing for another breath. It was a relaxed grin that paved the way for him to open up.

I interjected, "Do you think Shishang would like to join us?"

"Oh no…Shishang can't do that…he is very shy…pathologically introverted, you know?" Jun revealed matter-of-factly as he struggled to push air out of his lungs.

That would explain the furtiveness I picked up as Shishang crept about the apartment. I was now more curious than before about Shishang and wanted to understand the dynamic between them…but I packed that thought away. I had a rhythm with Jun that I didn't want to interrupt.

Jun took another deep breath like a swimmer ready to dive into a pool and swim its terrible long length entirely under water, steeling himself for a tremendous test, not knowing how far he might be able to go. But, realizing at the same time that what remained of his life, in terms of time, was likely not long and now might be the moment to record his story. Jun found his resolve and dove in with a splash that no doubt surprised him. He was eloquent:

"My life is a story about belated self-discovery, a life postponed until it was really too late to live it. During much of my time, I never understood who or what I was…much less the meaning of my feelings…I felt abandoned by life. I know that sounds like I am a victim…but consider my experience and I think you might agree I am one of many who share a similar story. Now that I have discovered myself it is as if I have found the grave of an identical twin brother I never knew. It is the essence of bitter-sweet and gives rise to very conflicted feelings: on one hand I have some welcome resolution, yet on the other hand, that resolution holds a harsh answer to a life full of questions." Jun avoided eye contact with me as he spoke and he looked to his left at the yellowed photos, his chest heaved again as he drew another breath of oxygen. I glanced at the photos as he inhaled…some young people, some old people…all likely long lost family members and other loved ones. One photo in particular stood out: a balding middle aged man and a younger friend…I suspected it was Jun and Shishang in earlier days.

As Jun continued, he spoke iteratively, sequencing the milestones of his life. Afterwards he began to dive deeper and reveal the nature of the important relationships in his life. He did so at times, as if guilty, confessing and seeking some absolution or self-forgiveness.

"I was born in 1939 in the middle of the war with the Japanese. I haven't any memories of this time at least nothing concrete. Most of my earliest memories are years later and are of Mao and the founding of the State. It was a proud time; the war was over and the future, or at least the future we were told to believe in, was bright. In school, I was a diligent student and performed all my lessons well. I sang all the songs they taught us and I memorized Mao's quotes. My parents were proud of me but my memories hold an empty satisfaction with what I was doing. I loved the praise my mother lavished on me, but I found no real substance in much of anything. I was restless. My father, a professor, was distant and always absorbed with intellectual discussions among his colleagues over the implementation of Mao's ideology. Later, when I was 22, my parents suggested...or really arranged a marriage to a beautiful young Shanghainese woman named Danxing. I remember being so fond of her beauty, her skills in home management and her cooking. I was delighted to marry her and took great pride in our union, but in hindsight, I hadn't a clue what I was doing. Often I would sit in the chair of our kitchen simply admiring her as she worked. But after five years of marriage to Danxing, my parents began to ask probing questions about our lack of children: they were exceedingly curious and I of course was bewildered. I sensed that they thought I was not normal."

"Why was that?" I inquired.

"Simply because I did not know how to make children...my generation was sexually repressed. This had never been discussed, either in my family or in schools. And I did not have many male friends who might have told me rumors or stories about this or that. Kissing and holding hands on school grounds or in public was prohibited. One night, after some uncomfortable intimacy, Danxing asked me why I did not love her. I was profoundly sad and cried when she said this. But she continued and insisted that if I loved her I would swell and put a baby inside of her. Understand Ke, this was the first moment that I began to think...'yes...I am abnormal'. Danxing, to whom I was completely devoted, now also thought I was not a normal man. Out of frustration she would frequently remark, 'All men want to make babies with women...except you.' This left me at a precipice. My wife wasn't sure of me, I wasn't sure of me and my parents were not sure of me...I had very few alternatives and the best one at the time seemed to simply back away from the cliff, recoil and disengage." Jun exhaled forcefully then inhaled quickly so as to continue as rapidly as possible.

"So, shortly afterwards, I began to see a number of doctors in an effort to resolve my problem." Jun released another breath which sounded like sandpaper on wood. I noted that Jun consistently framed the discussion as "not normal" and "my problem". I didn't know if he was using these terms in an historical context or might still see the situation as his fault.

Jun continued, "One doctor explained to me the process men and women perform in order to have babies and at once...I knew that this was something I would never, ever be able to do. It seemed utterly foreign and unappealing. The doctors insisted the process was the natural way and prescribed herbal remedies and special diets to enhance my libido. Of course this was all a waste of money." Jun waved his hands back and forth, crossing them and uncrossing them in front of him a way that emphasized the impossibility of the act in question. He was simultaneously amused and irritated as he reported this.

Jun continued, but first he inhaled then said, "Then the last doctor I saw was different. He seemed to understand my problem in a way the others, with their sterile approach and fancy medical terms, did not. He was very kindhearted and compassionate in his questions. In retrospect, he may have suspected I was gay or he may have even be gay himself and sympathetic or just reacting like some kindred spirit...I don't know."

"I see. But Jun, you have a child. How did this come about?" I puzzled.

Jun answered me flatly, "I would like to be able to say to you that I overcame my reluctance to engage with Danxing and was cured...but this isn't true." Jun's short, plain, honest responses, like this, were becoming his imprimatur in our discussion.

"Please tell me what happened?"

"I loved Danxing and I wanted to please her and repay her kindness to me...and at the same time put an end to the incessant, shameful questions. I wanted children also...but understand that this was exasperating for me as well as for her and the rest of the family. I felt on trial. The only moments of peace I had were when I thought about that last doctor with his tenderness and empathy for me. One night, while I was lying in bed with Danxing as she fiddled about, I imagined I was speaking with him...my beautiful, understanding doctor. And to my surprise, it happened...I transformed Danxing into the doctor in my mind and the dreadful task was completed! Danxing, luckily, became pregnant", Jun exhaled a mighty breath discharging a secret he had harbored for half his life.

"Interesting..." I was astonished. I looked over my left shoulder to see if Shishang was at the doorway but saw no one. He no doubt knew this story well or at least I suspected he did.

"At this point," Jun refilled his lungs with canned oxygen, "Life took on a very normal and routine course. Danxing raised our daughter, whom we named Liu, and I taught art in school. Danxing didn't seem to mind that there was no more intimacy after that one time...after all, she had what she really wanted and was probably relieved not to fuss about with a man who didn't seem to be attracted to her." Jun concluded, "Danxing had her life and I had mine. We intersected with Liu."

"When did you get divorced?", this was one of the last areas I wanted to cover...other than Shishang...before I got to the health care issue if I got there at all. Frankly, given the chat to this point I could predict the difficulties they had.

"It was a quiet matter...the date isn't so important but I think it was 1995...when Liu was 25. Danxing was on her 3rd affair. I really didn't care, but for her self-respect and for Liu, it was best." Jun pronounced this bit of information very casually and he meant it. I think it was a relief for him to be out of such a fiction.

"So, that really brings us to the modern era...so to speak", I euphemized with Jun.

"Indeed" Jun agreed then exhaled with a painful looking rasp.

"Maybe you could give me a bit of an insight into your becoming self-aware of your sexual orientation?" I thought it was time to get into the thick of things.

"Sure. But there was never really one particular 'A-hah moment'. It was a very gradual discovery. Ever since the beginning with Danxing and those excruciating moments in bed, I knew I was different but the magnitude of exactly how different was something I did not appreciate. I often thought about the time I was able to conceive with Danxing and the infatuation I had with the beautiful Doctor. I initially found that conflict puzzling but years later as more Western literature and newspapers became available; I began to learn more about homosexuality. At first it was something that I could not admit to myself, of course, but isn't that how we humans work after all? The truth demands to come out sooner or later...we can only keep things suppressed for so long. And I certainly kept it suppressed for quite some time. But after decades of clues, not just my failed relationship with Danxing and the Doctor's kindness, but the fact that I found male company enchanting and that with females merely filial, was too much to ignore." Jun went on like a defense attorney, detailing the facts, arguing the law and insisting his client was not just innocent but normal despite popular opinion to the contrary.

"By the time I discovered Danxing's second affair, I could only hope that she would divorce me and allow me to live in peace..."

"But Jun, why didn't you simply divorce her?" I asked.

"Two reasons" Jun explained. "First, I loved her and couldn't bring myself to ask her this...I didn't have the courage. Second, I wasn't entirely sure I was gay...and in those solitary moments when I thought I might be gay...I wondered...if I reconciled and admitted this to myself, what would I do next? I didn't know what to do about being gay even if I were single. Where would I go? I certainly wasn't about to announce it to my family...back in those days the local Magistrate might have found it his duty to subject me to a "healing process". There was really no definition for gay lifestyle at that time here in China. It wasn't as if in 1990 there was a huge community that offered support for older gay men. So I was stuck...it was a dead-end for me."

"So...is there a community for you today?" I shrugged my shoulders a bit prompting more from Jun.

"Hold on...so, I postponed...1985 became 1990 and her second affair came and went and her third arrived in 1995. By then things had changed a great deal in Shanghai and I was more confident...although a lot older by then. I had also ventured out and made friends who were similar to me and...I met Shishang. But to answer your question, at the time, there was no community for aged gay men. And there still isn't one now."

Ah, Shishang, I thought…now was the time I was going to learn about this enigmatic figure. I asked, "How did you meet him?"

"It was a though group of men who I found indirectly through the art community here. There was a lot of self- awareness happening…a lot of openly gay men. It was a new, wonderful world for me but one that I was on the fringe yet again. Most of them were in their 20's and I was nearly 60. Shishang was an art student…informally…who had come to Shanghai with his sister. He had an unpleasant life in rural Henan province and was essentially escaping."

"…Unpleasant how?" I asked, wanting particulars.

"The details are sketchy…but when he was 18, Shishang had been arrested for the theft of some small amount of food or something. His penalty was very harsh and he was sentenced to a prison for a year. While incarcerated, he was beaten, raped and castrated by a gang…", Jun spoke of Shishang's travails without much detail…trying to get passed this topic quickly in a way that seemed more out of respect for his friend than from a lack of knowledge.

"Hmmm…," I twisted my head in an attempt to show Jun I was listening attentively but said nothing…I was speechless.

Jun nodded, "Ghastly, I know…but true. Consequently he is very afraid of strangers…especially strange men. But he is warming up to you, I can tell." Jun tried to reassure me about the 'strange men' comment.

He continued. "After Danxing and I were divorced, I became immersed in the emerging gay community and grew close to Shishang. We moved in together in 2001…ten years later in 2011 I was diagnosed with emphysema".

"Ok…so this is where the story finds its connection with my book. Can you tell me how you cope with your illness?" I needed to get to the core as I had been with Jun now for 3 hours this day.

"I rely on Shishang for most everything. He cooks, cleans and cares for me. I saw a doctor two years ago and Shishang took me. But leaving the apartment even for small errands with him is a painful drama so we usually have everything delivered. So I will remain here in this apartment until I die. I don't want…can't leave Shishang alone."

I asked, "Have you explored a nursing home?"

"A few years ago…yes. But for a few reasons that isn't a realistic alternative. First, some nursing homes don't want or outright prohibit gay couples. Second, even if we pretended we were just friends, we would likely not be given a private room as most homes have 6 or more beds in each room. And that wouldn't work at all for Shishang given his condition…he would be transferred to the psychiatric ward. And that, I think we can both agree would be a terrible thing for Shishang. There are some new places that do have private rooms but we can't afford that. Moreover, I am done with pretending. Living as I do now, here in this apartment and dying in this chair, is what I will do."

"But Shishang will be alone when you die, no?" I wondered.

"Ke, maybe…maybe not…I cannot dwell on this. Shishang and I must live each day as it comes…We cannot dwell on how this story ends…we must enjoy what we have here and now", Jun declared.

"I understand. So, Jun, from your experience nursing homes will not allow gay couples?" I asked.

Slightly exasperated, Jun explained, "Oh, I really can't tell you the official policy at all…I do know what I have been told that is we wouldn't be accepted in the two that are nearby. We have lived together for 15 years...I don't want that to change and neither does Shishang...not for anything and certainly not because a care home won't allow us or accommodate us. And even if they did, imagine how we might be ostracized by others of my generation if they discovered us? Things have changed here in China...but mostly for the younger generation. We are comfortable here, together."

Immediately as Jun said those final words, Shishang, a tall thin, pale man of about 65 years, appeared at the room's entrance. His presence was solemn, almost like a monk, and he looked up only to glance at Jun. His emergence was a bit startling, but I noticed Jun's nod and Shishang quietly approached the recliner. Shishang was dressed in a long, faint purple silk gown tied with a yellow ribbon around the midriff, which made me think of the elegant dresses worn by concubines in the Tang Dynasty. Around his neck he had a small piece of chartreuse jade attached to a thin silver chain. He quickly passed from the hallway and sought protective refuge behind Jun's large chair. The pleats of Shishang's dress opened slightly with his movement giving the impression he was floating across the room. He stood now safely behind the chair and in what was more an affectionate gesture than a necessary one, Shishang leaned over to adjust Jun's oxygen tube. Jun lifted his hand affectionately and Shishang gently received it between the two of his. Again, Shishang leaned over Jun and whispered in his ear so silently I couldn't make out a single word. A few seconds later, Shishang straightened, and skewed his sight to the yellowed pictures on the table, avoiding any eye contact with me. His presence wasn't uncomfortable at all; rather he simply projected submission.

Jun took a breath, "Shishang would like to know if you want tea?"

"Hmmm...no thanks...but that is very kind of him to ask", I hesitated thinking that maybe it would be better if I should just accept. I was struck by Shishang's courage to enter the room with a stranger present, he was clearly a bit frightened.

Jun continued, "Shishang also wants to thank you."

Puzzled, I asked, "For what…?"

Jun breathed deeply again, he was tired. He said, "Shishang says you have helped by allowing us…me…the space to speak about our story. He is very appreciative of your efforts."

"Well…you're welcome…I don't know quite what to say…" I was surprised by Shishang's indirect yet very frank communication towards me.

Jun interrupted me, "Please, simply allow Shishang his gratitude…that is who he is."

At that moment, Shishang summoned up every molecule of fortitude in his slim frame, lifted his gaze and looked at me with eyes darker than a moonless night; eyes that dammed a universe of fear and pain. And then for a split second his face brightened with a forlorn smile; I felt like I was being pardoned. My understanding of Shishang expanded exponentially in that moment. Here was a man, who suffered unspeakable horrors and in return for understanding, a safe haven and I imagine, love, has devoted his life to caring for Jun. His unbounded kindness was unlike anything I have ever witnessed. There was a profound tenderness on Shishang's part that I did not expect; in fact I imagined he would be hostile. Instead, Shishang provided an environment which accommodated as near a normal life for Jun as he could have any legitimate right to expect. Nevertheless, Shishang remained a paradox and I think the only person that truly understood him was Jun…The walls that guarded his heart and soul were high and well-fortified.

Shishang diverted his eyes once again. He had communicated all he was prepared to with his glance. His appearance, however unusual in the robe, had gravity unto itself and made an unambiguous statement: "There. I am who I am…no apologies…nothing less and nothing more…with all flaws and managing as best I can with what I have. Now…please inquire no further." It was a look which conveyed an ultimatum and a defensive, fragile warning.

A moment of quiet passed again as I attempted to resolve the mystery that was Shishang. I felt it was time to go, so I spoke up, "Gentlemen…All good things must come to an end and this is where I must leave…"I wanted to make a very polite exit so I added, "I am afraid I have overstayed my welcome." I stood up and Jun immediately struggled in his chair. Shishang, with all his attentiveness, supported Jun as he adjusted himself in the walker. Jun was tired and I was afraid I had exhausted him.

I approached Jun to shake his hand. Alarmed, Shishang swiftly darted away to the side and without ceremony disappeared into the hallway, his gown fluttering from side to side, as my proximity to him grew uncomfortably close. No further glance, no more smile…Shishang was gone as quickly as he appeared.

"Jun…" I said and shrugged my shoulders in an apology to Jun for scaring Shishang, "I want to thank you for this opportunity. I wish you good luck and please thank Shishang as well. He was brave and…" I searched for an appropriate compliment, "…and, uh, very elegant in his purple gown."

Jun looked up at me with frosty eyes full of cataracts and simply responded, "Yes…Shishang is at times courageous and",…Jun paused as he passed by me and into the hallway. Then, looking back at me he finished his thought, "…and, well, lavender is indeed his favorite color. Ke, I hope you have found what you were looking for."

I followed Jun as he pivoted his walker and began the slow shuffle, banging away down the hallway. Once at the door, he stopped and turned to me one final time, "Ke, in my dreams, I am a kind and forgiving Emperor who is tolerant of everyone and every life, who lives for a century and is loved by his people, full of benevolence and reigning in a land where no one is made to feel abnormal or unwelcome." Jun raised his hands in front of him; palms turned upwards indicating a true and heartfelt statement.

I smiled at Jun...in a way not surprised at his musing, "That's a nice dream Jun, perhaps you will be that Emperor in the next life?"

"Yes and it can't come soon enough" Jun murmured in a wistful conclusion to our meeting.

"Goodbye Jun", I said, doubtful I would ever see him or Shishang again.

Jun closed the door as I walked down the hallway. I could hear that familiar twist of metal locks while I waited in front of the lift. The elevator came and delivered me to the lobby. I returned to the outside world, once again meeting oppressive heat, noise and pollution; it was late afternoon. I thought of Jun and his devoted Shishang as I walked down the street to the subway, a couple whose lives full of heartache and pain, I sincerely hoped might end with a modicum of calm and satisfaction. But I had reservations.

On a chilly winter's day six months to the day after my interview, the Emperor Jun passed from this life into the next. As he shut his eyes for the last time, safe and protected in the concubine Shishang's embrace laying together on Jun's chair, he drew his final labored breath and receded forever into his familiar dream. Shishang, dressed in his flowing robe, lowered his head so his cheek rested on Jun's brow, and whispered into his friend's ear, "My beloved Master...welcome to the Lavender Dynasty."

Author's note: 3 weeks after the death of Jun, I received a message from Jinsong. Sadly, tragedies sometimes beget tragedies and in Shishang case this was certainly true. Bereft and with no living commitment, Shishang saw little meaning in life without his friend. The morning before, Shishang woke up and could find no possible way to continue; his only alternative was exit. Slowly and deliberately, he dressed in his flowing purple silk gown and tied the yellow ribbon firmly around his breast. To his collar he pinned an old photo of Jun, applied a delicate cerise lipstick and donned his favorite jade necklace. He passed through the apartment, gently touching Jun's chair...bidding farewell to all the memories of the only purposeful life he knew. Resolved, he threw himself out the window of apartment 1704, ending everything.

The Chinese version of this story was translated from English by Sherry Xu

Jun and Shishang - Allocation of 9 Essential Relationships

Jun

Has	**Negative Transition** →	**Has not**
Self-Respect and Dignity	Healthy Body	Sufficient Wealth
Healthy Mind and Spirituality	Independence and Courage	Productive Engagement and Community Support
Happy Heart and Love		Reliable Friendships
		Strong Family Bonds

Shishang

Has	**Negative Transition** →	**Has not**
Healthy Body	Happy Heart and Love	Sufficient Wealth
Healthy Mind and Spirituality	Self-Respect and Dignity	Independence and Courage
		Productive Engagement and Community Support
		Reliable Friendships
		Strong Family Bonds

Discussion:

Jun: Jun was a proud and honest man and my conversation with him was profound. He spoke to me during our interviews as he had never spoken and I am grateful to have recorded his story. I believe that had Jun not been so ill, he and Shishang would have continued to live, possibly for another decade. But only possessing three Essential Relationships and with two in Negative Transition, his time was limited.

Shishang: My time with Shishang was limited having only met him for a brief moment. My distributions of his Essential Relationships above are inferred. Shishang's demise is largely a consequence of Jun's death as he was basically a healthy man of only 65 years. Prior to Jun's death, he had four Essential Relationships. But with Jun gone, Shishang could not withstand the loss of two of them; he was simply too fragile.

Jun and Shishang's ordeal has led me to think that the transition of two or more Personal Relationships is a difficult event from which to recover, especially since they each only possessed between two and three Essential Relationships.

"...for what remains of her life."

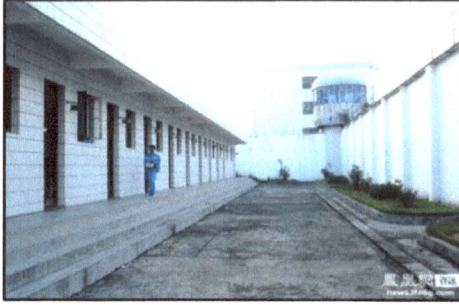

August 1963:

Song Wei slammed the small drinking glass down on the table. He was exhilarated...this was his 6th shot of Moutai that evening and he swallowed it in a single gulp. Wei liked Moutai[3]. But more than the taste, he loved the sense of accomplishment it brought and the way he could float above all his problems while he drank. The sorghum-sweet taste lingered on Wei's tongue as his mind drifted randomly through the day's events. Picking over his pork and rice with a pair of bamboo chopsticks, Wei lifted the ceramic bowl, shoveled food into his mouth and began chewing. At that moment his destiny arrived at the tip of a 5 inch pork knife. The blade was violently thrust into his thorax between the left scapula and the 5th vertebra, about 6 inches below his shoulder. It first cut through the soft cotton fibers of his shirt, then easily pierced the epidermis and sliced through the rhomboid muscle. The alcohol dulled Wei's reaction and before he could turn, he spat a mash of partially chewed food.

---

[3] Moutai is a sorghum-based, clear alcohol drink popular in China.

The strength behind the blade persisted and forced it past the 6th rib, ripping into his left lung. With a final shove, the black handle, soft and worn with years of use came flush with his back; the deed was done and Wei's fate sealed. Now horribly aware he had been punctured, Wei became frantic and struggled violently lifting his arms up, grasping wildly at what had penetrated him. But as Wei raised his arms, his scapula forced the knife down further, slicing down into lung tissue, tearing apart vessels. Blood poured from severed veins onto the left lung. Wei's long arms flailed, desperately reaching behind to remove what had impaled him. On his last attempt, Wei's right hand found the knife's black handle. He pulled up with a desperate intensity that drove the blade tip down, slashing the lung open further. He released his grip on the handle and collapsed onto the cold kitchen floor, cracking his head on the wooden chair next to him as he fell. Lying on the tile, he convulsed. As he shook, pinkish-white foam exited from his mouth and nose. He could no longer take a full breath.

His eyes bulged and stared across the floor at nothing as images of his life passed before him; first memories of his childhood and the brutal beatings administered by his mother...then as an adolescent, recollections of being chided mercilessly by bullies on the playgrounds of Jiashan...these pictures tormented Wei. His mind then fell upon his marriage to Xiaohong and a final sense of remorse was his last thought as darkness closed around him; he had no peace. He choked and shook again. With a lung nearly full of fluid, his torso shuddered as he exhaled his last breathe... Wei was now dead.

Wei's assailant stood motionless...then calmly stepped over his corpse and sat down at the table dispassionate and expressionless. She felt nothing; her only thought was time...all that remained was empty time.

November 1963:

Magistrate Weng Lo opened his court at mid-morning in usual fashion. First, the typical patriotic verses were repeated then a brief outline of the day's agenda. Earlier that morning his brother, Weng Shi, a local baker, had sent his son to Lo's home with a dozen fresh pork pies. Lo was particularly fond of this treat and his brother, younger than he by 4 years was a talented baker. His nephew, Weng Shi's son, arrived at Lo's home beaming and proudly presented the cakes to his uncle...the important Magistrate. Weng Lo loved his nephew as he had no children himself; Lo had promised his brother to assist his son and help him advance. He recognized a native intelligence in his nephew as having potential far beyond a simple delivery man. Despite being the Magistrate and all the import that this post carried, Lo's greatest influence was with the local Army division; but the vision in the boy's left eye was damaged which prevented him from a military career. Lo thought he was still suitable for a court appointment. Before he began with the case load, the Magistrate opened the bamboo tray and offered each of his colleagues a fresh pie.

Third on the agenda that morning was a notorious case. It was a murder. After conferring with his Surrogate, the Magistrate Weng Lo of the Glorious Court of People's Justice donned his spectacles and spoke gravely, "The criminal Wang Xiaohong shall stand and address the court. You are granted an opportunity to speak in your defense...proceed."

Wang Xiaohong rose meekly, cleared her voice and spoke. "Your Honor, I am guilty of my crime. I have no defense except for the fact that I do not recall the episode."

The Magistrate shot back at her impudence, "Failure of memory is not a defense under law. The court recognizes your guilt in this matter. What hangs in the balance is the severity of your punishment, indeed your life."

Magistrate Lo measured his words carefully, "The court advises you to offer your story in this regard."

Bowing her head, Xiaohong breathed deeply, "I am grateful your Honor."

She began calmly:

"April 16, 1951 was a brilliant, fresh spring day and I was the happiest girl in Jiashan. I knew I would be married to a handsome, rich, young man from a well-known family and be the envy of all the girls in the village. After all, my future was now secured. My best friend, Zhang Jian was elated for me. I remember of all the gifts she gave me, she was most happy of the small red notice which she took from the community board earlier that week and placed in my hand. It was the notice of a recent declaration from the Great Leader who had set a new law establishing the equality of man and woman in marriage. Yet, I didn't care much for wealth or security or woman's rights. I was unconcerned with possessions and wanted nothing more than to nurture a husband and have a family of my own. My parents often told me, of all my wonderful traits, my greatest gift was in seeing past a person's present troubles and find enduring value in his core. This is true, for better or worse. I didn't believe there was any such thing as a bad person or an irredeemable character flaw. I was, and am still, a small woman with a big, forgiving heart. My parents made a big deal over Song Wei's fortune, but I didn't care. I was wholly absorbed in the love I felt for Wei and trusted his guidance explicitly."

Xiaohong continued parsing through her memory:

"From the instant I awoke that morning, I was breathless and thought of nothing but my Groom. For me, he was a quiet, shy person with a penchant to become excited at times. I reasoned this was his youth and ambition but I was committed to him and supported my husband-to-be. I loved the tall quiet boy that he was; dutiful to his parents and studious in school. I recognized that he was less than social with other people, but this didn't matter to me. I understood that he was a homebody, having grown up largely in the courtyard of his family's home with little playtime among other children. I loved him blindly and accepted him gratefully as my husband with all faults, those known and unknown."

"For my parent's part, they spent months in long negotiation with the Song family doing everything they could to secure my union. They argued my beauty, provided examples of my industriousness and could readily prove my dedication to communist party dictates of deportment. Wei's family did not object in principle to our marriage though they drove a hard bargain. Wei once confided in me that, in secret negotiation amongst his clan that his family admitted I was a good catch for him. They felt he was quiet and reclusive and had an odd temper at times. They calculated that I would be good for their son."

"The hold out in the Song family was Wei's grandmother the Matriarch, Jiang Jie and to some extent his mother. Jiang Jie was a stoic and unforgiving person protective in every manner imaginable of the legacy she had helped create over the past 85 years. She outwardly questioned my commitment to Wei and cast doubt on my fertility. All she wanted was a male heir to her legacy. Jiang Jie remained unconvinced despite her son's argument that the modern era was upon them and her grandson, Wei, was capable of managing me. This appeal fell flat as Jiang Jie scoffed knowing full well the personality of her grandson. To her sensibility, she knew Wei to be an erratic child even if he were 23. In the end the Matriarch never openly consented to the marriage, she could not lose face in this matter. If nothing else Jiang Jie knew when to take a loss and move on. In this matter she merely argued less vociferously."

"In the days prior to the marriage, my parents had cleaned their home completely in anticipation of welcoming Wei's family for a visit. They bought me a new dark blue Zhongshan[4] with a matching cap. I recollect admiring its stiff, dark blue canvas fabric, so practical in every way. I was sure it would last 20 years. My parents sacrificed everything for me. The day arrived and Wei's parents hired a carriage to transport us through the village; the first stop was to my parent's home where we knelt at the entrance and bowed reverently. We then stood and toasted my parents who congratulated us sincerely. I was elated and Wei always smiled at me. We had a proud future, full of promise and happiness."

"During Moon Festival later that year, Wei and I had our first bad episode. Of all the holidays, I love this time of year as it meant that my family would gather and a joyous, reflective time would ensue. Yet this year, I was apprehensive. My uneasiness stemmed from the anticipation of questions about children...the ceaseless inquiries...the prying questions...all poking at me wondering why I wasn't pregnant. I reasoned with them that these things take time and biology cannot be rushed. But my heart suspected otherwise and I found myself providing half-truths to my family. Wei was oblivious to our difficulty and had over the past few months been concerned only with business. He was also drinking heavily."

"On this day, I think it was October 3, I remember he was light hearted and began his celebration earlier than usual with a round of drinking among neighbors. I was busy in the kitchen, chopping and carving meat for that afternoon's meals and could hear Wei's deep voice toasting with his friends and laughing heartily. It pleased me that Wei was happy."

"Later that day, Wei had the local bakery deliver fresh moon cakes to our house. As I sat at the table with our guests, Wei opened the door to pay the delivery boy and stumbled. His movement threw him off balance and he collided with the young boy holding two bamboo platters full of warm cakes.

---

[4] A Zhongshan is dark suit with a Nehru style collar. It is made of durable cotton twill and often blue or grey in color, utilitarian and popular during the Mao era.

The force of Wei's weight was too much for the boy and both hit the ground hard. The desserts scattered over the stone entrance."

"Wei was furious and shouted, "Clumsy Pig!" Wei began to fight with the boy swinging wildly. He punched the young boy in the head, near his left eye, splitting the eyebrow open. The blow cracked the knuckle of Wei's index finger. Wei shouted bad words and was thrashing the young man with his fists. I ran from the dinner table to the door and found Wei still striking him wildly. The boy was bleeding profusely from cut above his eye. I was begging my husband to stop, apologizing again and again."

"I had never seen a fight and the sight of my husband ruthlessly beating the boy made me vomit. At first I didn't recognize Wei, I thought it must have been some other man. I was…I was so confused. I grabbed Wei by the arm, then by the shoulder, his shirt, his hair. I was desperate to stop him. This was a moment in time that defied my reality and suspended everything I had known to be true about Wei. The violence was revolting…I did not know how this could be my husband."

As Xiaohong spoke, Magistrate Lo's ears shot up. He straightened in his chair and immediately recognized this story. His nephew's left eye had been damaged in a fight while delivering moon cakes ten years ago. His nephew refused to reveal who was responsible and the matter could not be pursued. Weng Lo checked his calendar to make sure the dates coincided and indeed, Wang Xiaohong referenced the exact same time as his nephew was beaten. Magistrate Lo did not believe in coincidences. Now, Xiaohong's story was instantly more complex than he initially thought. He knew the prominent Song family well and never suspected Song Wei was responsible for beating his nephew. With this revelation, the Magistrate's initial favor for the victim and sympathy for the Song family was now mitigated.

Xiaohong raised her hands, palms up emphasizing her bewilderment and continued:

"Finally with my mother's help, I managed to pull him off the boy. Wei crawled inside as my father stepped over him and went out the door. Once outside, Father knelt down beside the boy, gently attending to his lacerations with the cloth from the moon cake tray."

"The boy was hurt badly so my father gave him some money and told him to leave and keep quiet. Wei continued to curse and demand an apology from the boy; he was irrational. Our dinner was over…ruined by my husband's outburst. I had no explanation to offer my family. I just had to ask them to leave apologizing for Wei."

The Magistrate listened attentively, completing a picture in his mind that had puzzled him for a decade. Xiaohong closed her eyes for a second, collected her thoughts and continued:

"After this incident I attempted to discuss the situation with Wei. I wanted to understand why he exploded but he refused and didn't want to speak with me. He receded into himself and rejected my approach. I reassured him I loved him no matter what but he would not hear me. This was a turning point as if something awful inside had awoken and seized control of him. I can say he never was the same afterwards."

"Then, in the Spring Festival of 1954 he disappeared for 2 nights. First, I remember he came home from his parent's factory drunk…he changed his shirt and left. He never said a word to me. I asked him if he wanted dinner but he ignored me. I had prepared a feast and he just left. Not a word, not even a glance. He just closed the door behind him and walked away. After the first night, my best friend came to pay me a visit and said her friend saw Wei across town with someone. She didn't know who but it was a woman. His manager at the factory was a nice woman and I figured he must be doing some work with her. When he returned home I did not ask him about it…we just carried on. I wasn't sure what to do so I tried to be as normal as possible. In the next few days he was brusque with me in our conversations…he had a temper and was short…lacking patience with me on everything."

"After Spring Festival, our lives fell apart rapidly. Our relationship was the complete opposite than it was when we were first married. Two months later, in the early summer, I came home and found Wei in our bed…in our bed…with another woman. I…I was stunned and outraged at the same time…that he had not only broken his faith to me but chose to do it openly and…and…in my bed. I was deeply insulted and hurt…he had no right. *NO RIGHT!* I shouted at him and told him to get out and take his whore with him. He slammed the door and got dressed with her. I left the house and went to my friend's home for the rest of the afternoon. But I did not tell her what happened. I was embarrassed and ashamed. I felt it was my fault but I did not know what I had done to cause this."

As Xiaohong spoke these words she was out of breath recalling the wretched details with the same shock that haunted her 9 years ago. She looked about the courtroom, first to the left and then the right, at the men and women gathered together as she described those shameful moments; it was obvious to all she was a woman spurned in as harsh a manner as one could imagine. She had no reason, no logic for the trespass. But more than the shame of the violation, more hurtful than the dishonor, more than anything was the ignominy of the humiliation she endured in the days and weeks afterwards. Xiaohong didn't need to tell her friend what was wrong; Jian knew. And as the secrets of life go, it wasn't long before the whispers of Xiaohong's tribulations grew into popular village folklore.

Xiaohong pressed on:

"In the late summer of 1954, I pledged to myself to move on with my husband and forget this ugliness. I had faith I could rehabilitate our marriage…I just needed to commit myself more completely and show Wei I was dedicated to him. To demonstrate my allegiance to Wei, I made delicious dinners for him, I kept the house clean every day, I worked to prove to him I was worthy of being his wife and he shouldn't dismiss me. Yet the more I worked, the more he escaped into his affair. The more I attempted to build a comfortable, forgiving space around us as husband and wife, the more he grew angry with me."

"About a year later, Wei began a new phase of vile behavior. I had decorated the house for Moon Festival. Wei was drunk when he came home. I asked him to join me for dinner but he wouldn't come out of the bedroom. He was in a dark non-communicative mood; his work had not been going well and he was borrowing money from everyone. I begged him to come to the table and eat. When he didn't respond I went into the bedroom and confronted him. As I demanded a response, Wei slapped me. I fell back against the chair and collapsed onto the floor. My arm throbbed in pain and I could not raise myself. Wei stood above me, his fists clenched and simply warned me to leave him alone. He said, "Do not tell me what to do...I am tired of your pathetic efforts in our life." Wei then walked out of the house. After he left, I simply lay there on the floor for hours. I began crying, in part because my arm hurt badly, in part because my husband had hit me...and I had never been hit before. I recognized then that I was failing as a wife."

"Wei never again brought the woman back to our house, but his affair with her became widely known. People would speak about him and his sordid behavior behind his back, but never openly as his family controlled so much of the city's affairs. What did continue were the beatings. He would disappear for a few days, return to the house and hit me...that is...if I had healed from the last beating. If my arm was still in a splint, or my leg bandaged, he would spare me. But I could rest assured that the next time would be equally as savage and unrestrained. He enjoyed administering pain...punishing me for something...I didn't know what. And nothing would stop him while he hit me. I would implore him to calm down, promise him anything if only he would cease. No entreaty mollified him…he had so much anger. While he hit me he would always blame me for his misfortunes…whether it was his business or other things…I was culpable for everything…he held me responsible for anything he chose."

The Magistrate searched his memory and recalled having heard something of Song Wei's anti-social behavior. But as a matter of course, Weng Lo did not trade in gossip. He was a judge and was tasked with measuring crimes against the law then administering appropriate justice.

Xiaohong was staring at the Magistrate as she began the end of her statement:

"Then a few years ago, I heard that the woman he was carrying on with left him. I am not sure why…I did not inquire. But it was at this point that Wei's depravity assumed a dimension which I never thought any person was capable. One evening, it must have been in the summer of 1960 or maybe later, Wei came home early and drunk as usual. I was not expecting him as he rarely came home so soon and dinner was not yet prepared. This infuriated Wei and he hit me twice. I ran into the bedroom to escape him but he followed me and hit me a few more times while I lay on the bed, all the while shouting how useless I was. He then suddenly stopped and looked at me. His eyes burned with resentment and he smelled foul. He placed his hand on the neckline of my shirt and in one motion ripped it apart with such force that the buttons flew off. He then stripped my pants off and I knew he was going to rape me. Beating me was no longer sufficient. He needed to find another outlet for his violence. Wei forced himself on me and did what he wanted…I initially tried to repel him but he wrapped his large hands around my throat and threatened to kill me if I resisted. But he wasn't done…raping me was still insufficient and didn't satisfy his hate. No, after he was done, he dragged me by the arm into our small courtyard, threw me onto the stone walkway where he once beat that poor young boy years before and then...proceeded to urinate on me. I fell onto my back, closed my eyes and as he sprayed me with sour pee. I wished that I were dead. Wei had become vicious, degenerate and immoral. He was now thoroughly irrational...and I could not find a way out of this predicament."

On hearing this, the Magistrate looked about the courtroom and took note of the disgust on people's faces. He then glanced at his Surrogate who appeared equally revolted.

Xiaohong kept on:

"This conduct was the new normal for Wei. My husband would come home after work and two or three times a week, he would beat me, rape me and then urinate all over me. When I was adequately defiled, he would stop, go back into the house...then eat and drink more. I desperately wanted to rid myself of Wei...cleanse my life of him and rinse the memory of Wei away forever."

Despite the brutality to which she had been subjected, Wang Xiaohong lifted up her head and looked straight at Magistrate Lo...not out of any conceit but with a look of basic human pride that said to everyone in the court, *'I erred...I know...and I will receive my punishment as you deem proper...but everyone has their breaking point...this was mine.'*

"That, Magistrate Lo, is my story," with this Xiaohong ended simply. Her demeanor throughout her statement was without fidget. If nothing else, her soft voice rose and soared above the court with clarity and truth...she told a story that had the ring of authenticity. With her conclusion finished, the Court's official observers shifted uncomfortably in their seats and the public onlookers began gossip; some whispering the word 'execution' while others revealed their uncertainty and speculated vocally about acquittal.

The Magistrate paused for a moment, stunned by the whole of what he had heard. He wasn't certain what to ask Xiaohong next. Lo removed his spectacles and rubbed his eyes. He looked back at Xiaohong and asked her, largely out of curiosity, "Is this why you killed Song Wei?"

Xiaohong answered, "I do not remember the actual moment I killed him. But I did. I murdered him because I could no longer live like an animal. I loved Wei with all my heart and I did everything I could to support him and be the perfect wife. I allowed him to brutalize me...I did anything I could for him and to find a way through our hell together. In the end, I could no longer endure my own subordination. My subservience was an attempt to rectify our marriage and it was the wrong approach...it made him worse. I failed Wei...and allowed him to grow into a monster. And then, when I could no longer tolerate the monster, I killed it. He was a victim of my shortcomings as a spouse."

Xiaohong's statement resonated in the ears of the Magistrate. He reflected that she was in full possession of her act, however wrong and however corrupt. After she spoke, Xiaohong, in only the second display of emotion that day, buried her face in her hands and sobbed heavily.

The court fell silent. Magistrate Lo shuffled papers, turned and conferred with the Surrogate. Xiaohong's sentence was his domain exclusively but he was expected to seek advice from his assistants. The Magistrate spoke to his Surrogate and told him he felt there was sufficient evidence to convict with a death sentence. But, Weng Lo, in the same breath said that he, as a judge, was offended by the victim's repulsive behavior and felt Song Wei was somewhat responsible for his own murder. The Surrogate praised the Magistrate's wisdom and concurred as he usually did. Weng Lo did not mention his earlier discovery; the realization that he had a connection with Song Wei though the attack on his nephew and could substantiate depravity and violence of which Xiaohong spoke. As he thought to himself he measured Xiaohong's experience, the impact of her statement and...the irreparable injuries suffered by his brother's son. He could not dismiss the weight carried by the sum of these facts. They all pointed to a very bad person: Song Wei. Nevertheless, Wang Xiaohong, the Magistrate concluded, must be held accountable for her crime.

Magistrate Lo was ready and spoke loudly, "The criminal Wang Xiaohong will prepare to receive her sentence."

Before Xiaohong could wipe her tears away Magistrate Lo began...

"Wang Xiaohong, the Glorious Court of the People's Justice has found that you have committed the heinous crime of murder with reckless abandon, brought scandal upon your family, the village and deprived your in-laws of their son. You are morally corrupt and dissolute. Confess your crime to the People, now!"

On cue, Wang Xiaohong raised her red, swollen face and lowered her hands. She stared ahead and said obediently, "Magistrate, I am guilty of this crime."

The Magistrate folded his hands on top of his desk, leaned forward then began again, "Wang Xiaohong, you are wicked and your debased criminal act deserves the punishment of execution. The Song Family accepted you as their daughter and you repaid them with the murder of their son."

The Magistrate took a breath then began again:

"The People are offended by your corrupt morality. However, this court also finds sufficient evidence that your crime was not wholly of your intention; it is acknowledged there were external factors to your debauchery. Therefore, the punishment of execution is suspended and the People sentence you to prison for what remains of your life. You are hereby remanded to the custody of Jeng Do Prison for Female Criminals."

Magistrate Lo sat back in his chair, sounded the gavel with a satisfaction rare in his experience. Full of self-approbation, he seldom had administered justice so soundly; two wrongs righted and mercy shown.

April 1964:

Three months after her trial when Xiaohong was 39, she was formally admitted to Jeng Do. The Warden issued her a uniform, recorded important personal information and received those items, wedding ring and bracelet, which she would no longer require. The process of stripping her former life away was in process, they would be sold to defray the costs of her incarceration. Her hair was cut short above the ears and she was given an antiseptic shower. Later that morning, after the administrative work had been completed, Xiaohong was taken to her cell. Her home from that moment forward was a small 3 square meter cement room with a square window at the top whose thick opaque glass allowed light or dark only. There was no view possible.

Xiaohong entered the cell and sat down on the small rug that would serve as her mattress. In her lap was a bowl and wooden spoon, issued to her by the Warden. She was allowed to retain a small cardboard box which held a faded notice given to her before her wedding by Jian and a note written to her at the end of her trial by her mother and father. The iron-gate shut and was locked by the guard and she walked away. At once Xiaohong was alone, the stillness of the cool prison air and the silence of her cell had a finality that was reassuring. She thought, "It is all over and I am at peace. I will now go to sleep and wake up when I am 95 years old, just before I die. These years will pass in an instant and my crime will be settled by forfeit of my life."

Xiaohong never read the note from her parents as she knew it contained bitter words of disassociation. She couldn't brook their disappointment; her own disillusionment for the way she failed Wei yielded enough regret for her life. She knew they were angry with her for what she had done and the dishonor she brought to their lives not to mention economic ruin at the hands of the vengeful Song. She did read the faded notice that Jian had given her on the wedding day, remembering how excited her friend was about the note's news. Jian told her the Great Leader had ensured all women a new, safe future. Xiaohong unfolded the note and read it for the second time in her life. It contained the words of a new legal decree by Chairman Mao which Xiaohong found ironic. The notice read:

Article 1: The feudal marriage system based on the arbitrary and compulsory arrangements and supreme act of man over woman, and in the disregard of the interests of children, is abolished.

Article 2: Bigamy, concubinage, interference in re-marriage of widows, and the extraction of money or gifts in connection with marriages, are prohibited.

She mused to herself, 'Equality under the law is wholly different than equality under the roof'. Xiaohong folded the notice and placed it back into the box thinking she would miss Jian greatly. She regretted the embarrassment she may have caused her and hoped she would live a happy life.

May 2015

Wang Xiaohong still lives to this day in a small cell behind the secure walls of the recently rebuilt New Jeng Do Prison for Female Criminals. A wizened old lady of 93 years; she is a model prisoner and exemplifies corrected behavior. No one at the prison today was there when Xiaohong arrived in 1963, she has outlasted them all. Her record is clear: She stands as a reminder to the younger inmates that the system works and one's crimes can be atoned with proper focus and dedication. There is no doubt she has been rehabilitated. But after 52 years of incarceration, she is thoroughly institutionalized having had little interaction with the outside world during this time. At this point, no life for Xiaohong would be possible beyond Jeng Do. But then, none of what occurs beyond its high walls matter. All that is relevant is attention to daily routine and steadfast commitment to reform.

In 1972 she received notice that her father died. In 1980 Xiaohong was informed that her mother passed. She places these notes into her cardboard box. It has become a depository for a history she has all but forgotten; it is evidence of a time she isn't sure existed. In those moments of daily life, when something triggers a distant memory she regards it as pre-history, a preface to her real life in Jeng Do; a safe, predictable life where she has found purpose and meaning.

Luckily, Xiaohong has been in fair health most of her time in Jeng Do, at least no health issue has terminated her life to date and that is an accomplishment in itself. The budget at Jeng Do for surgical procedures or other special medicines often necessary for the elderly is non-existent. There is no dentist, no ophthalmologist, no cardiologist and certainly no geriatrician. The costs for such specialists are the responsibility of inmates' families. But Xiaohong has no more family. In 2008, she became aware of a lump in her abdomen which has since grown to the size of a grapefruit. Nothing more is known about this condition, other than it impedes her stride and slows her routine. Recently, her eyes have gone weak and her stomach is frequently upset. With no relatives, she must rely on the benevolence of volunteer organizations who contribute items to prisoners; unfortunately no one donates surgery. Those with whom she is closest are her imprisoned friends and jailers; the latter are as kind to her as one expect them to act towards a non-threat. They often refer to her as grandma. But they can't shrink the bloated tumor in her gut, clear her cataracts or calm the burning acid in her stomach. These ailments go unresolved. Care for the aged in prison, any prison for this matter, in China or in the West, is sorely lacking.

Xiaohong was born an altruistic woman who longed to devote herself to another, build a family and live as happily as she possibly could. She is a selfless, noble human who naturally placed others, their feelings and their needs before her own. Her personal desires were always secondary and acknowledged only after others were content. Long ago Xiaohong accepted her fate with ineffable Taoist conviction; she is a consequence of her own design and solely responsible for her situation. The question of 'what if' serves no purpose and simply doesn't occur to her.

Nevertheless, her compassion and goodwill have risen to the surface. During her time at Jeng Do, she has inspired her fellow inmates to something greater than themselves. Consequently, they now define one another in terms of accomplishments rather than their verdicts. For three decades after she was sentenced, Xiaohong taught the other convicts important skills such as reading, sewing and calligraphy. But today she is retired though many Jeng Do women still seek her advice and consul; she is the sage among them. By sheer dint of example, Xiaohong has created a culture of kindness for these women and instilled in each of them hope for the future. She is a living legend and the heroine of Jeng Do.

But Xiaohong has always eschewed accolades. Over the years she simply carried on each day with her chores, quietly and obediently. Xiaohong has always been Jeng Do's wash woman and cleaned her fellow inmate's clothes dutifully. Every day, all day as the weeks turned into months, the months passed to years; she scrubbed the spots that stained and rinsed away the accumulated odors of Jeng Do. When finished, Xiaohong would wring the foul water from the garments and carefully hang the clothes to dry in the cleansing sun as if she were rectifying their crimes as well as purifying her own. So far, a 52 year penance of ablution...and still counting...for what little remains of her life.

Wang Xiaohong - Allocation of 9 Essential Relationships

Has	**Transition**	**Has not**
Self-Respect and Dignity		Sufficient Wealth
Healthy Mind and Spirituality		Independence and Courage
Productive Engagement and Community Support		Happy Heart and Love
Reliable Friendships		Healthy Body
		Strong Family Bonds

Discussion:

Despite the calamity that is her life, Wang Xiaohong is at equilibrium. She lives in a very stable environment; one in which her four remaining Essential Relationships will not likely change. But her health is another matter, something which she has little to no control over given her living environment. In so long as her health is not terminal, the consistency she has in daily life will sustain her for a long time. I can imagine her dying a natural death; one that isn't accelerated by the Negative Transition of any Essential Relationship.

Wang Xiaohong's story is a good example of how sustaining Interpersonal Relationships can be and their importance in the absence of Personal Relationships.

Like Mother, Like Daughter

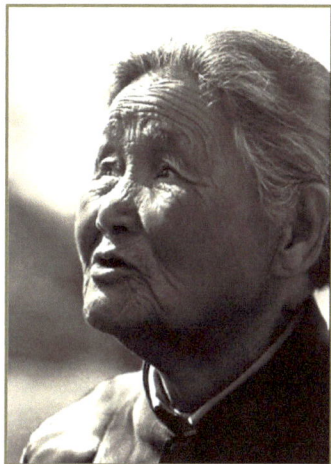

In the appendix of this book is the reprint of a story I wrote for my first book, "Enter the Ageing Dragon". It is an interview actually, of a discussion I had in 2011 with a young woman I called Jiang who worked in a nursing home in Beijing. During our chat and without much prompting on my part, she revealed the gritty realities of being a migrant worker and other heart wrenching aspects of her life. Jiang disappeared after I interviewed her; she just picked up and left her job like migrant workers often do...always looking for a better job and more pay. Jiang's story was captivating in many ways and I have wanted to speak with her again, if for no reason other than social curiosity, kind of a longitudinal study of sorts. However, I have been unable to find her. She disappeared into the masses and is lost among the multitudes of transient workers roaming the ranks of menial labor. The nursing home had no further information on her whereabouts, no forwarding address, nothing. So, in a final attempt, I resorted

to the information about her home town in Chongqing which she gave me during my interview. I discovered that I had a fair amount of detail about her family's location...not a specific street address but a neighborhood and other details about stores and restaurants which gave me some reasonable hope that I might find her or a clue to her whereabouts. Armed with this information I set out to find Jiang or some trace of her. This story is the surprising conclusion to Jiang's odyssey.

*Before you proceed, if you did not read the first interview with Mrs. Jiang's daughter, **you should stop now** and read it in the Appendix.*

Bishan is a small, hilly city north of Chongqing by nearly an hour's drive. I was in central China on some business and Chongqing was a short detour west from my location. Once I finished with my obligations, I caught a short flight and was on the ground, in a car, headed north to Bishan in less than 90 minutes. I arrived around 11:30am, reviewed my notes and began my search, knocking on doors in the general location indicated by Jiang's description. I spoke to a lot of strangers that morning each one simply closed their eyes and shook their heads dismissing my inquiry regarding their familiarity with Jiang or the whereabouts of her family home. After three long hours, I began to lose my enthusiasm for this mission. I pledged to spend another hour after which I would return to Chongqing and schedule some business appointments for the remainder of the day and tomorrow before I had to leave. My next seven queries were a bust, a mix of empty stares and brusque no's. However, the very next person that I ran into claimed she was Jiang's aunt and directed me to the family home. I was stunned and flooded with enthusiasm...I picked up my pace and trotted down an alley and across a small foot bridge following the woman's directions exactly.

When I arrived, in front of the house identified by the person claiming to be Jiang's aunt, I found a plump, old woman dressed in loose fitting pajamas and plastic slippers sitting on a stool cleaning cabbage. Every line on her wrinkled face told a story of some past pain; a raw, purple bump on her forehead oozed a clear fluid. She ignored me as I stood in front of her so I spoke up and said 'Ni hao'. I introduced myself and asked if this was the home of Jiang. The old woman looked up at me, stopped her cleaning, squinted and simply said "No...This is my house. I am Jiang's mother. She doesn't live here any longer." She returned to her cabbage.

I felt for sure I would now find Jiang; I launched into an explanation of who I was and why I was there.

My discussion with Mrs. Jiang begins as we sat in the small entryway to her modest one room apartment, containing a bed, table, two chairs and a stove all crammed into 30 square meters, set on an alleyway in a western Bishan neighborhood. The doorway was just a few feet from the road...so close in fact that I wondered if a motorcyclist or motor-cart might crash into us at any minute as we sat in the entryway:

Bromme 柯博明: Hello Mrs. Jiang. It is nice to meet you finally. I am quite surprised to have found you.

Mrs. Jiang: Greetings Ke Dong. This is an unusual situation and the last thing I ever expected today.

<<Mrs. Jiang smiled and bowed her head slightly as she acknowledged me>>

Bromme 柯博明: As I explained to you when we first met a few minutes ago, in 2011, I met you daughter. She was working at a nursing home in Beijing and I was writing a book about the development of the senior care industry in China. We had a good discussion and she told me many things.

Mrs. Jiang: She is a smart girl Jiang! Was she an important person in the facility? A manager maybe..?

<<Mrs. Jiang was on the edge of her seat with these questions excited to learn what her daughter had achieved>>

Bromme 柯博明: Well, no. She was not a manager. But she was, and is I am sure, a hard worker...learning a lot every day. In the book, I recorded my discussion with Jiang and it became well known as a sober description the nursing home industry in China and its workers. I...

<<Mrs. Jiang interrupts me, claps her hands together...and exclaims...>>

Mrs. Jiang: I knew Jiang was going to be famous someday!! She is such a good girl and smart too!

Bromme 柯博明: Yes, well...I agree. Jiang is a good person. Mrs. Jiang...I was hoping to learn from you where I might find Jiang. Do you know her whereabouts?

<<I tried to gently reel in Mrs. Jiang. I wanted to stay focused on finding her daughter>>

Mrs. Jiang: I see...No Ke Dong...I don't. I have not spoken to Jiang in years. You are the last person that I know who saw her.

<<Mrs. Jiang instantly turned worried>>

Bromme 柯博明: Really? Based on what she told me of your relationship, I would have thought the two of you to be in close contact. Jiang had a phone and so do you, so...

<<This was not good news...Jiang was very emphatic about her closeness with her mother>>

Mrs. Jiang: We are close...we have always been close. But when her father returned home, I don't think she was happy about that. She hasn't called in a long time. She changes her number frequently.

<<Apparently, Jiang disappeared again>>

Bromme 柯博明: Mrs. Jiang...your daughter told me a great deal of her troubles at home when she was young. Why did Mr. Jiang come back?

Mrs. Jiang: Jiang told you about the family?

Bromme 柯博明: Yes.

Mrs. Jiang: He ran out of money...this is his home also so I cannot keep him away. Listen Ke Dong, my daughter had a hard youth and was exposed to many difficult things. Maybe I am to blame for it, but these were my decisions at the time. Can you help me find her again?

<<Mrs. Jiang looked down at her trimmed vegetables as she spoke these words. Her demeanor became slightly defensive>>

Bromme 柯博明: I don't know Mrs. Jiang. I have nothing really to go on. It seems an impossible task. All my hopes to find her were with you. I wanted to speak with her again for another story in my new book.

Mrs. Jiang: Of course...if I hear from her I will tell her you are looking for her. She may not call after so long.

<<We both paused for a bit. I wasn't sure of what to say next>>

Bromme 柯博明: Mrs. Jiang, do you mind if ask you a few questions?

<<With little to go on at this point I decided to learn more about Mrs. Jiang>>

Mrs. Jiang: Please go ahead. Will I become famous also?

<<Mrs. Jiang's spirits lifted. She and Jiang shared the same wry smile>>

Bromme 柯博明: Hah ha! You seem a great deal like your daughter. Who knows, maybe you will be famous. When I spoke to Jiang back in 2011, I was clear about the fact that I was going to use our discussion in a book I was writing. I promised her I would not use her name or anything else that identified her. She agreed to speak with me on that basis and, of course, I kept my promise. I came here hoping to find her or at least a way to find her because I wanted to continue her story. Now, that isn't possible...but I am thinking that maybe you might offer an interesting perspective on her and your lives together. Would you be willing to chat with me?

<<With her simple, honest responses, Mrs. Jiang did indeed remind me of her daughter. But as the discussion continued I became more and more aware of an important distinction between them. The generation that separated them as well as the new China/old China dichotomy, was as wide as an ocean>>

Mrs. Jiang: I guess so...Sure!

Bromme 柯博明: Thank you. When I saw Jiang she was 36...today she would be 41. What is your age, Mrs. Jiang? And Mr. Jiang?

Mrs. Jiang: I am 71. Mr. Jiang is 69.

<<Mrs. Jiang tossed a trimmed head of cabbage into a basket which held other cleaned vegetables>>

Bromme 柯博明: How is your health?

Mrs. Jiang: I am fine.

<<Mrs. Jiang was nonchalant to the point of indifference>>

Bromme 柯博明: Forgive me for saying, but you don't look fine. You look uncomfortable and that bump on your head is bleeding.

Mrs. Jiang: I am 71 years old Ke Dong...an old woman. What do you expect? I fell off my scooter the other day and scrapped my head.

<<I saw no scooter anywhere near her small house and I doubted she could ride one in her condition anyway. I noted that Mrs. Jiang's definition of old age was 71 years.>>

Bromme 柯博明: Ok...But please take care of that bump, it looks bad. Does the doctor say that you have any health problems?

Mrs. Jiang: I promise...the hospital says I have a sugar problem. And Mr. Jiang has a fatty liver.

<<Mrs. Jiang was very casual about this. Her swollen limbs and face indicated diabetes. Mr. Jiang, it seems has hepatic steatosis...and probably hepatitis C. Both illnesses will likely end in their deaths if left untreated for much longer. The life expectancy for urbanized women in China is 76; for those in rural areas it is much less>>

Bromme 柯博明: I see. Do you take any medication for your sugar problem?

Mrs. Jiang: No.

Bromme 柯博明: And what about Mr. Jiang...does he take medicine for his liver?

Mrs. Jiang: Who knows...

<<As she said this, Mrs. Jiang shrugged and chopped the stem off a head of lettuce with a short, ill-tempered stroke>>

Bromme 柯博明: Mrs. Jiang can you also tell me what you do these days?

Mrs. Jiang: I cut vegetables for the restaurant next door and do other jobs. Anything I can do to make money.

Bromme 柯博明: And Mr. Jiang? Where is he?

Mrs. Jiang: Drinking no doubt. He will be home when he needs to sleep or eat.

Bromme 柯博明: I see. Does he make money to help with the house expenses?

Mrs. Jiang: He has a small pension but not much...certainly not enough for all his cavorting.

Bromme 柯博明: He is a pretty old man to cavort...no? If I might ask, why do you support that?

Mrs. Jiang: Well, it is better than the alternative. Men cavort at any age...it makes no difference.

<<Mrs. Jiang is a woman, tried and tested for most of her life and under no illusions about her situation>>

Bromme 柯博明: What alternative is that?

Mrs. Jiang: Chaos...fighting...nastiness. I am too old to have that...so I ignore it...and him.

<<Mrs. Jiang tossed another cleaned cabbage into the nearby basket and picked up one more>>

Bromme 柯博明: So, Mrs. Jiang, let me understand. You have a sugar problem, you husband has liver disease...neither of you take medicine for these conditions. You both have small pensions but it doesn't really cover what you need so you work and Mr. Jiang doesn't. If you don't mind my asking how much longer will you live here?

Mrs. Jiang: Until I die...Where else would I go?

<<No illusions, indeed>>

Bromme 柯博明: Of course, Mrs. Jiang...this is your home.

<<Speaking to Mrs. Jiang about senior care facilities seemed more than absurd. There was no way she would even consider such an arrangement...and why should she?>>

Mrs. Jiang: Yes it is...

<<I felt like an intruder...so foreign and so far from her reality. But I was grateful for the moment to for the glimpse she offered into her life and her plain, sentient responses>>

Bromme 柯博明: Here, please take my business card. My number is on the front. If you ever hear from Jiang, have her contact me. But let me ask you one last question Mrs. Jiang...Why do you think your daughter keeps on running?

Mrs. Jiang: Ke Dong, you are a smart man. She is looking for a better life. What is there for here in Bishan? She is unsatisfied with a life like I had...she is a younger generation and wants to be rich...she is simply different than me and has opportunities I never did...Can you blame her? Ke, if you ever see Jiang again...tell her that I love her...all my heart is with her for the future...that I wish her all the success she dreams of...that I am sorry for the way things worked out. But please, make sure she doesn't come home...it would not be good. I don't have much left in my life...as much as I would like to see her again...she cannot come back here.

<<What Mrs. Jiang said in these few sentences, she delivered looking past me and across the foot bridge to the neighborhood beyond. But in her last sentence, as she beseeched me to warn Jiang against returning home, she lifted her face up and stared into my eyes. A harsh life had injured her soul and jaded her perspective but when it came to Jiang; She was a mother whose love was limitless...her intent was pure and caring. The distinction between the two of them was as I had first suspected: generational and not so unusual.>>

Bromme 柯博明: I don't blame her at all...but why can't she come home?

<<Stupid question on my part>>

Mrs. Jiang: Please Ke Dong, just grant an old lady her wish...It costs you nothing so please tell her not to return home. She must live her life and purse her dreams without the burden of Bishan any longer.

<<I knew why but I wanted to hear more from Mrs. Jiang on this though she denied me. I suspected that Jiang and her father wouldn't have so much a reunion as they would a confrontation...which would benefit no one with its potential for violence>>

Bromme 柯博明: Ok, Mrs. Jiang...I will.

Mrs. Jiang: Ke, you should go now. Mr. Jiang may be home soon and I don't want him to find you here. I would not be able to explain without mentioning my daughter.

We said goodbye and Mrs. Jiang sitting there, quivering lips holding back a mountain of emotion, simply turned to her vegetables, picked up her knife and continued cutting and trimming; it was an obvious distraction from the welling up inside her. I picked up my backpack, left her front hall and headed back across the footbridge. I stopped on the other side, turned and waved to Mrs. Jiang. She waved back, then wiped her leathery face clear of tears and returned to her vegetables. In an hour I was back in Chongqing and the next morning I caught my flight and returned to Shanghai all the while regretting that some other ending did not occur, though meeting Jiang's mother was an event in itself. My job was done and although I had not found Jiang...I thought I had enough of a story to conclude, however simple it might be.

Two months later, I spent a Sunday writing the above interview in my office from the notes I kept as I sat with Mrs. Jiang. After I finished, I reread the interview, made a few edits and saved the work as final forwarding off a version to the translator so she could begin her work. I closed my laptop, locked my office and headed back to my apartment. Jiang's story was closed.

On Monday morning as I woke up I looked at my phone and parsed though the early morning messages: 12 emails from the US, 3 Wechat messages from friends and 1 text message in Chinese that I couldn't read. Ignoring it, I stretched for a moment then got up and prepared to work out; a breakfast at 930am meant both a short workout and a late arrival at the office. My breakfast meeting was with a prospective hire for a new program I wanted to promote later that year and for the upcoming Trade Show I run annually. I actually needed two new staff, a business development officer and an office administrative person. The office had gotten so busy that the office administrator was especially crucial.

I left breakfast and began the short walk to the office. As I walked, I forwarded to my Project Manager the Chinese text message I received that morning for translation. After a minute, she returned my note and said it was someone who knows me. The very next note from her said that the author of the text message was now in the office waiting for me. It was unusual and a bit unsettling; I hurried down the block, into my building, up the elevator and into my office. My Project Manager met me in the vestibule and said the person, a woman, was in my office waiting.

I opened my door and there, standing next to the window, as simple as I remembered her 4 years ago, was Jiang. Older, no doubt, but Jiang none the less.

I smiled broadly. We laughed out loud and both of us declared this a true surprise for each. I told her that I had just visited her mother looking to finish her story. We shook hands heartily and I offered her a seat. Jiang replied that she had, quite by coincidence, called her mother last week and wanted to tell her she was ok and looking for a job in Shanghai. When she called her mother, her mother told her that I had been looking for her to finish a story. Mrs. Jiang gave her daughter my contact information…and warned her not to go home. As Jiang told me of her conversation with her mother tears streamed down her face. She knew exactly why she couldn't go back though she wanted to see her mother badly. I also told her of her mother's wish…for her not to go home…but that her mother asked me to tell her that she loved her very much. I gave these words to Jiang and she lowered her head into her lap then looked up and thanked me. She said her mother never said those words to her, but she knew them to be true.

We sat and spoke for about an hour as she told me where she worked for the past few years, where she had been, etc. She also said she had been taking some study courses at night to learn business. Obviously, she was trying to improve herself and move ahead. I was enormously proud of her.

Below is our conversation after the pleasantries of meeting again were finished:

Bromme 柯博明: Jiang, what are you going to do now that you are here in Shanghai?

Jiang: I need to find a job. I came here because my boyfriend has a construction job for two years...but I need to work also. I want to get my mother out of Bishan and bring her to Shanghai so I can keep an eye on her.

Bromme 柯博明: That is a very loving idea Jiang. I remember, when we first spoke in 2011, you said you would care for her when she got old.

Jiang: Yes, I really want her to be in Shanghai with me.

<<At that moment and with those words I had an avalanche of thought. I then acted mostly on inspiration but also partly with sympathy for Jiang which I have carried since the day I met her>>

Bromme 柯博明: Jiang, I have a need for an office administration person...would you like to do it?

Jiang: Really? I don't know, Sir...I think it is too hard for me.

<<Jiang looked astonished. This was no doubt the last thing she had expected this morning>>

Bromme 柯博明: Don't be silly Jiang, of course you can do it!

Jiang: What do I have to do and how much do you pay?

Bromme 柯博明: I want a full year commitment, you cannot disappear...that must stop. You take care of the office, support the marketers and sales people, order supplies...and I pay a lot more than an aide in a nursing home!

Jiang: I see...Thank you Sir...I am so happy...I want the job!

<<*Jiang clapped her hands together enthusiastically*>>

Bromme 柯博明: You are welcome Jiang...I am happy for you...I will hire you.

Jiang: But Sir...what about your story...my mother said you wanted to finish the story from before. I came to help you finish...don't you want to finish?

<<*She was so eager. I paused for a moment and realized the saga of Jiang had come to a happy ending*>>

Bromme 柯博明: Yes...Jiang...We just did...

<<*Jiang sat for a second thinking and then smiled brightly*>>

> *Authors note: Two months later, Mrs. Jiang stepped off a China Eastern flight from Chongqing and into the welcoming arms of her daughter; they are now finally reunited. The two of them, along with Jiang's boyfriend, live a happy, simple life together. Jiang has made good on her promise to care for her ageing mother.*

Mrs. Jiang - Allocation of 9 Essential Relationships

Has	Positive Transition ←	Has not
Independence and Courage	Self-Respect and Dignity	Sufficient Wealth
Healthy Mind and Spirituality	Happy Heart and Love	Healthy Body
		Productive Engagement and Community Support
		Strong Family Bonds
		Reliable Friendships

Discussion:

Mrs. Jiang is a lucky person and she has her daughter to thank. While in Bishan, Mrs. Jiang's future looked bleak as she only had two Essential Relationships; it was an unstable existence in every respect and likley not to last long. But the reunion with her daughter, Jiang, has enabled Mrs. Jiang the retrieval of two Essential Relationships. I would expect Mrs. Jiang to enjoy her daughter for a long time to come.

Among all the profiles, this is the first example of a Positive Transition of an Essential Relationship. There remain a lot of variables in Mrs. Jiang's life, not the least of which is her troubled relationship with her husband, but I think it is clear that the important aspects of her daily existence have improved dramatically.

LONGEVITY TREE by Raymod Li

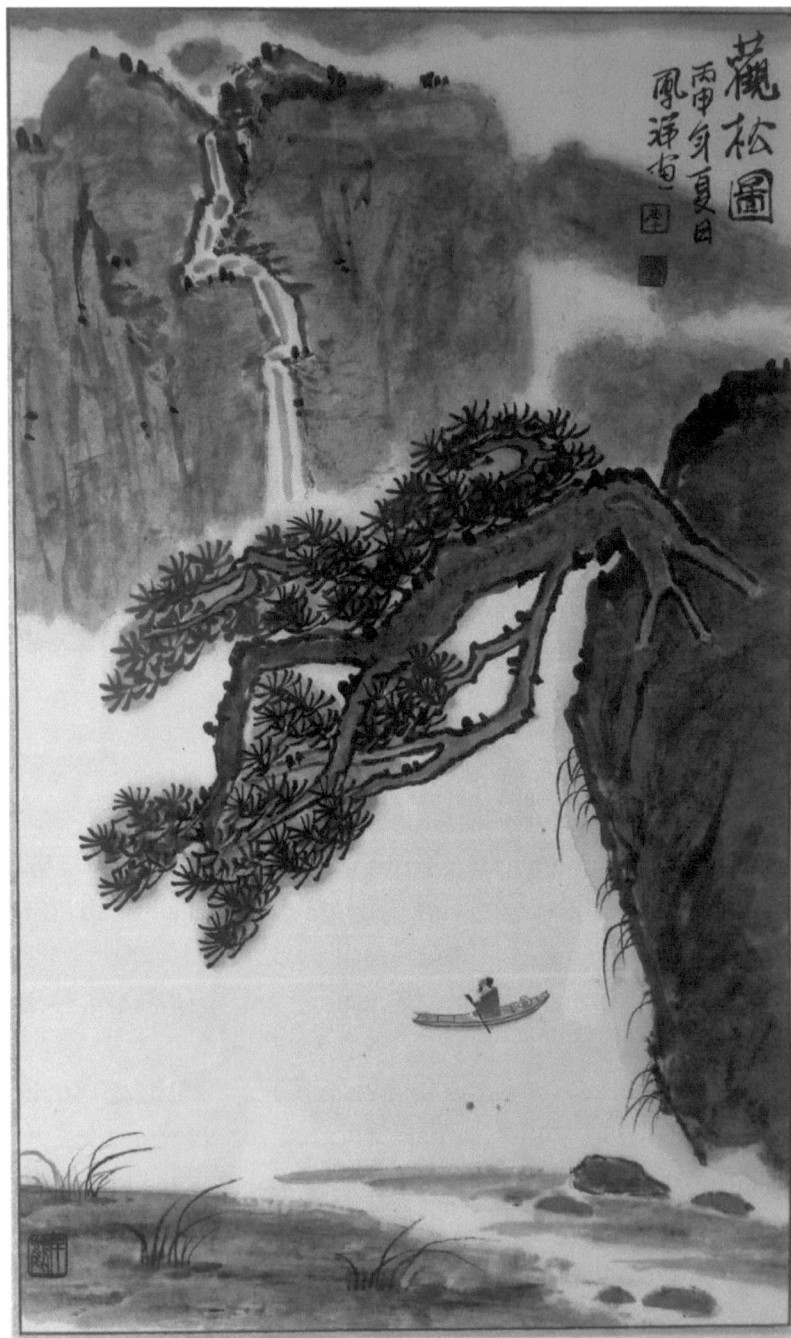

A Beautiful Voice

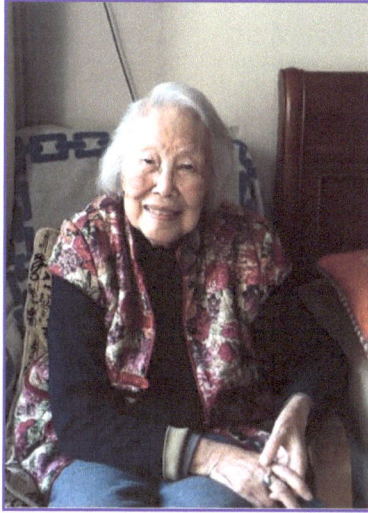

Su Xiu[5] sits in her chair, composed and self-assured yet her face is soft and sweet. I have just arrived at her apartment and introduced myself; I can see immediately that she radiates a life full of experience and satisfaction. I have come to speak with her as I have heard that her story is remarkable. I am sitting directly across from her as we speak and her answers are clear and honest. As we progress into our chat, she is amused by my questions. She expects me to ask her only about her career as China's most famous voice-over artist. Mrs. Xiu was China's dubbing queen. She remarks that everyone who interviews her wants to know about her life in film. But I am less interested in her professional achievements than I am in learning about how her experiences earlier in her life have determined her destiny. I want to know the intimate details, especially those vulnerabilities that confront

---

[5] Su Xiu is her real name and this is her picture. She wanted to be present for this interview. However, I have used a different name for her husband.

her today as she ages. I also know that her husband died about ten years ago and his passing was traumatic due to dementia.

Xiu is 96 and a thoroughly enchanting woman. She is elegant, delightful and in relatively good health albeit a bit infirm though her mind is sharp. As we begin our chat my initial suspicions about her are confirmed. I learn that Xiu has led an extraordinary life, full of rich experience, intrigue and self-fulfillment; she is a blessed woman. As she speaks, I enumerate her gifts in my notebook: she was the wife of a devoted husband, the mother of three talented children who in turn presented her with 4 grandchildren, a gifted entertainer whose adoring fans praised her one of the leading stars of China's early film and radio industries.

After 30 minutes, I am done gathering the fundamental facts of her life. She was born in 1926 in Changchun, to parents originally from northern China; they were both teachers. Her father lived to 102 and was born in 1885. Her mother passed much earlier. Incidentally, Su Xiu is the first person I have met whose parents were born prior to the bloody Tai Ping rebellion and had first-hand experience of the Qing Dynasty's decline along with the chaos that ensued. She is in many ways, a door to a fascinating history, not just her own. Su Xiu never finished university for reasons I will explain later, but this isn't all that relevant. Given her natural beauty and sublime voice, she gravitated from radio to China's nascent film industry which consisted mostly of imported foreign films. As she engaged more and more with the circle of artists enthusiastic about film, her career took shape and her destiny was set. She was the lead female Chinese voice in such famous western films as Dr. Jekyll and Mr. Hyde, The Red and the Black and, most notably, Driving Miss Daisy.

Mrs. Su sits in her chair eager to answer my questions. I want to know about her husband so I begin:

"Mrs. Su...please tell me how you met your husband, Ji Yu?

"I was beginning my studies in education in Harbin and I loved watching sports. Ji Yu was a basketball player...so strong and tall. I loved watching him direct the team, running around the court and scoring points. He was so athletic", Mrs. Su is love-sick with the memory of her husband. She continues, "One day I interviewed some of the players for a newspaper article. I asked him what he liked most about the sport."

I was curious, "What did he say?"

"He said he loved the tactics of the court...and since he was tall...he had a natural advantage. The game came easy to him. This was true...he was so rhythmic and much better than the other players", Su Xiu easily remembered him and especially that moment she and he first spoke.

"Did you fall in love with him immediately?" I ask, seeing now that Mrs. Su's story is indeed centering on her husband and their relationship.

"Oh no...not immediately...but quickly! He was so manly and I loved his voice, especially the way he called for me...there was such a gravity between us", Su Xiu describes her husband as one would expect...but the intensity that she conveys as she mentions the "gravity between us" is palatable. Despite the passage of time since his death, the bond between them has not weakened.

I am solicitous and want to encourage her further, "Please...tell me more about him."

"Well, he saved my life", Mrs. Su intonates heavily on the words 'saved my life' which in a very effective way, underscores just how grave the situation must have been. I was beginning to notice the way Su Xiu used language to emphasize her relationship with Ji Yu.

"Really...how was that?" I say.

"In 1941 he was an engineering student and transferred to Beijing to attend a better school. One day, after we had been in Beijing for about six months, I attended a conference on education. About half way through the meeting, the building was seized by Japanese troops. They announced through speakers that we were guilty of sedition against the Imperial Army and were now their prisoners. For some reason, they believed that the program I was attending was a Kuomintang gathering. They garrisoned about 50 soldiers in the building and separated the men from the women. The officers were harsh...barking out orders to their troops...marching up and down the hallways each hour...their leather boots stomping the floor and swords clanging about. I was scared and didn't know what was going to happen. One of the girls managed to escape, she told Ji Yu that I had been arrested and was being held in the school. We were kept there for a long time. On the afternoon of the third day, two Japanese soldiers came for me...I was panicked and my friends screamed as they dragged me away. I thought I was finished but they didn't hurt me....instead they took me downstairs and...I was astonished...Ji Yu was waiting for me in the lobby", Mrs. Su is still frightened by this event...she looks down and into her lap, wringing her hands together nervously, her face is white with fear as she understands the horrors that might have occurred...and did so to many other women.

I didn't have time to ask her what happened next when Mrs. Su looked back up at me, her dark eyes full of utter admiration for the person that was Ji Yu...she said, "He bought my freedom with the money that he had saved for school. Ji Yu compromised his future to save me...we couldn't stay in Beijing without money so later that night we ran away to Tianjin to stay with friends."

I breathed deep then said "...He loved you very much."

"I loved him very much...and when we got to Tianjin we decided to be together forever...we pledged our love for each other that night", as Su Xiu spoke, I was struck by her solemnity; I have seldom heard such earnest words. I sat in my chair imagining that moment 75 years ago: Su Xiu and Ji Yu, lying together on a makeshift cot huddled close together shielding each other from the cold Bohai Bay winds, their faces lit by a candle's flame, listening to each other as they took turns pledging an oath of eternal faith. It occurred to me their union was honest evidence that little else could be more powerful than love born during the ravages of war.

I wondered, "Did you get married in Tianjin?"

"Oh no...ceremonies were not possible during the Japanese occupation. So we just made our own commitment", Su Xiu shrugged her shoulders and smiled innocently.

Thinking out loud to Mrs. Su, I say, "That's possibly the sweetest story I have ever heard. So, when did you leave Tianjin and move to Shanghai?"

"In 1951, after the civil war[6]...I got a job in a radio station and Ji Yu got a job as an engineer. I was with the radio station for about a year when I was asked to do my first voice-over for a foreign film", her tempo picks up a bit. The previous discussion was heavy but revealed Su Xiu as a deeply sensitive woman.

---

[6] Refers to the war between the Communist and Kuomintang parties.

I remark, "That must have been exciting!"

Visibly enjoying a fond memory of a happy time for a moment, Mrs. Xiu exclaims, "Yes…for the next 10 years, I was popular and very busy."

"Why just 10 years? What happened then?" I sensed her story was going to take another unfortunate detour.

"It wasn't good. I was well known in the media and deeply associated with foreign influences. So as the forces of the Cultural Revolution gained momentum, they became suspicious of me and felt that I was a risk. So I was sent to a match factory in Jiangsu Province for re-education. My job was to cut wood", Su Xiu recounted this period of her life with angst and frustration…chopping sticks into little pieces must have been a mind-numbing, useless situation. For the second time in her life she had to manage the vagaries of a political machine, heavily armed with an ideological drive. I can only imagine the setback she suffered.

"How long were you gone for?" I asked.

Su Xiu paused, "…8 years." Her words came out, stained with a bitterness which imparted a clear sense that she had little use for this episode in her country's history.

"I see…that must have been difficult. You had to leave your children with Ji Yu?" I say, but want to avoid political discussions.

"Yes, he took care of them," Su Xiu murmurs.

I continue to speak, "Mrs. Xiu, after your husband's death you moved to Hangzhou. What did you do there?"

"When Ji Yu died, I could no longer manage by myself in Shanghai. I couldn't eat, couldn't sleep...I was manic", Mrs. Su lamented.

Su Xiu moved into her daughter's apartment in the spring of 2004, six months after her husband's death. She closed the apartment she shared with Ji Yu for 40 years and just left...leaving furniture and nearly all their personal belongings behind. She was in a rush to leave. The memories of Ji Yu haunted her...his wonderful smell...his clothes...his tall lean body...all of him still occupied that apartment and she couldn't bear it. Most of all, it was the grief of the last six years of his life that pained her the most. In 1997, Ji Yu developed Alzheimer's and by 2000 he was all but lost to her. He no longer recognized her and frequently referred to her as the "maid".

But as much as she felt the need to escape Shanghai and the rid herself of the constant reminders of his presence, Hangzhou was unknown, so unknown that she felt anonymous. And despite her daughter's presence...she felt more alone than in Shanghai. She was between two worlds, neither of which fit.

Mrs. Su continued to tell me about her time in Hangzhou, "I had settled in Hangzhou but I couldn't find my home there. I tried to cook, clean and do all those things that I loved doing for him...like wash his clothes and prepare the house for him. I tried to do these things for my daughter and she appreciated them...but it wasn't the same. I was not home."

"One afternoon, I was walking along the Xixi Wetlands pathways. It was early summer, but not too hot so I decided to take a long stroll. As I sat on a bench for a rest, I closed my eyes for a moment. And then...the wind picked up a bit and I heard him", Mrs. Su was deadpan serious.

"Heard whom...?" I asked.

"My Husband, of course," She smiled. Her face brightened and her natural red lips parted widely as she spoke.

"What did he say?" I was off balance a bit.

"This first time, he only spoke my name. I was startled and a bit afraid...but I knew it could have been no one else. His soft low voice was like a hug...I knew how he called me...it was him...I was sure", Mrs. Su was emphatic...absolutely convinced that Ji Yu's spirit was in the winds around her.

Mrs. Su continued with her remarkable story. For the rest of the summer she returned to that bench next to the river at the Xixi Wetlands. Two to three times a week after breakfast she would rush out of her daughter's house and walk as fast as she could to that bench. She would sit there and close her eyes, relax and open up her soul...waiting for more contact with her husband. At first, she reports it was a seldom occurrence, then as she gained a greater understanding of how to listen for him, he began to call more for her.

For a moment, Mrs. Su returns to the hard memories of caring for Ji Yu, "When I lived in Shanghai, I was afraid that I no longer loved my husband. It was difficult to take care of him and the worst part was he no longer knew me. Understand that he hadn't used my name for most of the 6 years he was sick. He had forgotten me. Every day, day in-day out and often times in the middle of the night I would wake up to attend to some issue he had. He would go for weeks without acknowledging me...and demanded that I sleep in the living room. But I understood...I knew what he was going through and my duty was to ease his suffering."

Su Xiu pauses then brightens, "But when I heard him call my name while sitting on the bench…I fell in love with him all over again…like the time I first saw him playing basketball and he spoke my name…his voice, that beautiful deep voice…It all around me again…I felt embraced. Now he was back and I spent hours at the bench speaking to him. I was so full of joy!"

"Did he respond when you spoke to him?" I wanted to know more about her conversations with Ji Yu.

"No…I would speak with him and he would simply say my name…then one day…he did speak to me." Mrs. Su confirmed then drifted off and looked winsome…gazing out her bedroom window.

I wanted to ask her what he said but I thought it might be too personal to do so. But after a moment of quiet between us I found the courage and asked, "Mrs. Su…Can you tell me what he said…do you mind if I ask?"

She returned from her far-away stare and looked at me as quiet and still as a statue. For a brief moment I could feel the earth spin on its axis while I waited for her to speak. When her words came, she spoke a declaration as if correcting a wrong. Her words underscored a sincere belief that she had truly connected with her husband…that they somehow managed to cross over the divide that separated the living world with the hereafter…that their oath of eternal faith made that cold winter's night in Tianjin transcended the real world and allowed them to reconnect.

Mrs. Su glanced out the window. She calmed herself with a breath and said, "I buried my husband then I left him…it was wrong of me. He had never forgotten me…certainly not in Beijing…but I held him responsible for not remembering me while he was sick and I shouldn't have been so harsh; he still loved me. He reached out to me and forgave me for leaving."

I pressed, "But what did he say exactly?"

She continued staring out the window, looking at the hills in the distance. Then those red lips parted, she turned to me and quietly admitted, "He asked me to come back home...He asked me why I had left him in Shanghai...why I moved away and left him alone." Tears streamed down her face as she recounted his words.

She took a full, deep breath...her chin quivering, eyes wet with tears and lips trying to form words...but no further ones came to her.

"When did you come back to Shanghai?" I was curious.

"Oh...it was too urgent to wait...I left that afternoon!...I took a taxi to the train station and was back in our apartment before dark. I called my daughter once I got home and explained everything." Mrs. Su was relieved, leaned back in her chair and chuckled at her own impetuousness.

"That is quite a story...Tell me Mrs. Su...do you still talk with Ji Yu?" I inquired.

Su Xiu responded to me without hesitation, "No...and I don't need to....we are together again. He is now at rest and I am at peace...happy once again in our home here in Shanghai." Mrs. Xiu folds her hands neatly in her lap and smiles. She is indeed content.

I review my notes briefly, and shuffle them back into my briefcase. Her journey is a wonder...and no matter the journey, whether real or imagined, she is as she says, "happy and at home". I stand up and thank her graciously breaking into a few slight bows at the waist. She politely dismisses my appreciation as if it is her exclusive honor to speak with a loyal subject. I bow again respectfully as one would to a real queen. She raises her hand and I receive it gently and kiss her wrist…I am bewitched.

Su Xiu - Allocation of 9 Essential Relationships

Has	Negative Transition →	Has not
Independence and Courage	Healthy Body	
Healthy Mind and Spirituality		
Productive Engagement and Community Support		
Happy Heart and Love		
Sufficient Wealth		
Strong Family Bonds		
Reliable Friendships		
Self-Respect and Dignity		

Discussion:

Su Xiu is an Essential Relationship rich person. One might have expected the loss of her husband to have been the beginning of a downward trend for Su Xiu. But her extensive network of both Personal and Interpersonal Relationships has more than compensated for this loss. Clearly her celebrity status and her unique abilities have contributed to her bounty, but from my interview of her, it is apparent that she has lived honestly in every respect. I suspect that, notwithstanding her increasing frailty, her Essential Relationships will sustain her for some time.

The Man from Exuberance

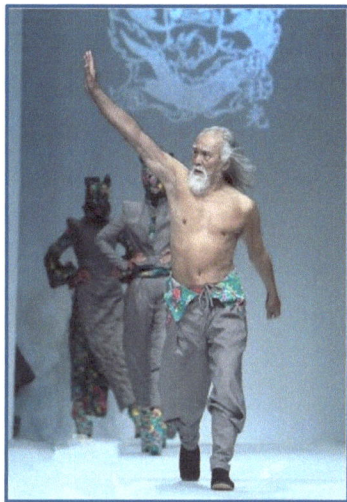

Behold...Wang Deshun! He is 80 years young. Wang's entire life has been a ceaseless pursuit of soulful understanding and artistic expression. For most of his career, he was a dramatic actor, sculptor, film star, author...and still is all of these in abundance. But today he is also a supermodel and aspiring techno-rock DJ, to the delight of the fashion industry and young audiences throughout China. The only indication that he might be more than 65 years old is his flowing white hair and beard..."Insignificant!", claim the bevy of young, beautiful women who share the runway with him, they adamantly declare his long white locks make him all the more attractive. The female models adore Wang. As he arrives for the fashion show they swoon about him and flirt shamelessly. They kiss him and drape their arms around his bronze, muscular frame like giddy school girls fawning over the high school quarterback. Then, Wang bursts into action on the runway; a humorous counterpoint to the stoic marching of his female partners. He is animated, kinetic...prancing about shirtless, waving to everyone in the audience, smiling, blowing kisses, and loving life abundantly; the crowd erupts with wild approval. In all seriousness, I wonder while watching the phenomenon of Wang: "All that remains is for him to strip naked and break out into a rap dance...I wouldn't be surprised." He is a rock star of sorts. The lead entertainer at any event, pleasing the crowd to no end...the outlandish costumes of Gorgio Armani pale in comparison to the Wang sensation! He is dearly loved and his zest for living is so contagious, so palatable that you want to be him and inhabit his energy. I am convinced that in a previous life he was a happy-go-lucky Italian fisherman living on a sun-soaked Mediterranean island, singing songs about making love with beautiful women as mermaids splash about, hauling in nets bursting with fish and...living life out-loud with reckless abandon.

But that is what Wang does...but who is Wang the man? Wang is a one man hit parade of joy and happiness; he is a curious creature...an improbable Chinese *bon vivant*, over-flowing and effervescent. His life stands as undeniable proof that positive thinking and a healthy lifestyle are essential ingredients for contentment not to mention long life. Of course, Wang is also blessed with superior DNA as good nutrition can only go so far. I met with Wang in his DJ studio recently and wanted to learn more about the marvel that he is; I had no doubt the conversation would be inspiring but I needed to know how he got to be the public Wang...what was his journey? More importantly, how is it that he is, at his age, so active and healthy? What element forms the cellar of his soul?

Through a friend who was once his art student, I scheduled a meeting, flew off Beijing and rushed into in a cab to meet Wang. I arrived and entered his music studio a few minutes before our scheduled chat...it was a hive of young, bohemian musicians buzzing around...in and out of spontaneous jam sessions, trading chords and riffs. The scene was cool, the energy was vibrant; the room was full of Chinese beatniks, the avant-garde of the local creative set. Wang saw me through the glass wall of his acoustic cell where he practiced cues and transitions for an upcoming DJ gig on the Great Wall. He opened the door and loud, throbbing electronica spilled out into the studio lobby...the bass pulsed so forcefully my heart was overwhelmed and jumped a beat. Wang removed his headphones, smiled and motioned through the music indicating that he would only be another minute; he shut the door, the music retreated and my heartbeat reset. I walked up to the thick glass window of the cell for a closer look. Wang's back is turned to me as he snapped his fingers with one hand and spun a turntable with the other...he shook his hips and mimed a dance while mixing tracks. I looked up at the LED TV screen above him...a composite of blinking lights and brightly colored information including volume levels and songs tracks. I did a double-take on the names...there was a furious energy in them: "Freight train in my head", "Make that shit funk", "Squirt you with my slippery body acid", and the exceedingly dark, "A+ Mother Fucker". I was completely bewildered...conclusions were impossible at that point except for the easy deduction that Wang has no barriers.

Minutes later a lissome Chinese young lady approached me; in a British accent she asked me to follow her to a room Wang had reserved for our chat. I soon learned her name is DJ QQ. She is Wang's eldest child and his muse as she is an accomplished DJ in her own right helping her father to learn the trade. But had she not told me that Wang is her father, I could have guessed; they are copies of each other. Like Wang, she is attractive, tall and has a personal gravity that presents her without a spoken word. Also, like Wang, she looks 15 years younger than her actual age. She was wearing tight jeans and a leather jacket, her long thick black hair cascaded down her back. Like a teasing veil, her bangs draped low over her dark eyes and when she blinked, her long eyelashes tangoed with her hair. That day, she sported blonde frosted highlights and black fingernail polish...all contributed to quite the hipster appeal; she carried it well...confident and smart.

DJ QQ offered me a seat, her warm Mayfair voice is polite but assertive, "Would you like coffee or tea?"

"Hmmm, coffee please…thank you!" I smiled…her gracious hospitality is exceeded only by her charm. DJ QQ turned, leaving the room with an alluring supermodel swing to her hips. She is 47, Wang is 80…they look 32 and 65, respectively. I am left thinking chronological age in this family is physically invisible and certainly has no bearing on the occupations they chose.

In short order, the door opened and Wang burst in…his face is electric and his smile is so moving I want to immediately stand and rejoice his arrival. DJ QQ followed her father into the room holding two cups of coffee, one for me and one for her; alas, Wang drinks only catechins-rich green tea. He reached out to me with open arms and warmly embraces me…as if he were my grandfather greeting me after a long absence. His familiarity is engaging…and his ease with me is comforting. Patting the chair next to him, he begged me to sit and relax.

I began by explaining that I want to know as much as I can about his life in the 3 hours he has given me. Wang nodded and started…alternatively speaking and stroking his long white beard in a quiet but dramatic fashion:

"I am the second oldest of nine children, born in Shenyang into a family so poor we were always looking for food. My parents were never at home…father worked in a restaurant and my mother always worked odd jobs. These were the early days of the war with the Japanese…and we had nothing…every day was a quest for survival. And because life was so difficult, I had no relationship with my parents as you might know such a relationship; basic human warmth…to mention hugs and kisses, never happened. The need to find food and subsist was the only thing that mattered...from my fourth birthday I had a job which consisted of foraging for my next meal...I would leave home early and return late. Dinners would consist of boiled water flavored with soy sauce and maybe a root...but not much more. I did not see my parents much: sometimes in the early mornings or late at night...that is if they were still home. Death and dying was all around us in those years. Nobody young today can imagine the horrors we endured; life today is a paradise compared to those times." Throughout his opening words, Wang's gestures pantomime the violent and the tragic.

Wang dispensed this history surgically and spoke these words for what they described...raw, unembroidered facts of his early life. It was what it was...he dealt with it...he survived...he moved on. As our chat progressed, two dominant themes emerged as consistent currents throughout his life: the struggle to survive and his quest for artistic expression. They have defined his life and framed his personality from his earliest experiences to his present endeavor as a DJ. But I sensed there was something else deep inside Wang that pushes him.

Wang's first real job after the troubles of his youth waned and the war subsided was as a bus conductor robotically collecting tickets from passengers and announcing each stop as the bus drew near. The monotony of making change was numbing for Wang, but again, it was a question of survival...he was making enough money to eat. So he pushed on, knowing that like the war, this too would pass and what comes after would be better. For the next 15 years, jobs came and went but it was the position with the *Wen Gong Tuan*, the USO version of the Red Army, which led him to his destiny. In the *Tuan*, Wang had the opportunity, at long last, to perform. He and his fellow troop members sang and danced for 7 years, performing for soldiers during lunch, dinner and weekends. But the playbill was written to support party ideology and the material was largely dry and artless.

Nevertheless, he endured, and again this reinforced the two essential elements that have come to characterize his life.

Luckily, Wang's time in the *Tuan* also brought him his wife. She was also member of the troop and they performed together for the entire time. Wang detailed the times they spent together in the *Tuan*:

"We fell in love while we were employed at *Tuan*. Performing together was so much fun even though the material was dull and repetitive. Each day we woke up and looked forward to seeing each other and preparing for the program the next day. We could not speak about our feelings but we recognized a mutual attraction; the rules governing us at *Tuan* forbid any relationships between actors. We abstained for 7 years...it was difficult. But the moment the Cultural Revolution was essentially over, we lunged for each other and DJ QQ was born 9 months later! Hah!" Wang rolls back in his chair and claps his hands joyfully recalling the moment. Listening to him, I understand at that instant he was set free, no longer a prisoner of artificial limitations. He could then begin to explore life and his passions...and he did just that.

For the next two decades, Wang was a fountain of artistic production. His work on stage gathered the attention of art critics from all over the world and they praised his creativity. Generally, he was seen as the leading avant-garde performing-artist in China in the 1980's. He traveled to Europe and studied mime with Marcel Marceau, performed vaudeville in front of Notre Dame and sang love songs for cash on the banks of the Danube. After returning to China, he produced a number of dramatic stage productions most notable of which, and receiving significant critical acclaim, was a "theater of sculpture" piece depicting the torrid love affair between Camille Claudel and Auguste Rodin. He was now fully engaged with his artistry. And today, 35 years later his dramatic performances continue. To be released in

June 2016, Wang stars in a dramatic Chinese film called "_Winter_", about a lonely old man who saves a little girl on the treacherous Snow Mountain.

Interestingly, my friend who made the introduction to Wang detailed yet another unusual occurrence in Wang's past that speaks directly to his repudiation of convention. As the story goes, Wang was teaching a drawing class and it seems he became frustrated with the students. They were hesitant to explore the human form with their art. Their initial sketches of a mannequin placed in the center of the class were lifeless, flat and rendered the human form mechanical. He would beg the students not just to draw but to feel the body under their pencils. "Let the body take form!" Wang would implore his students. Still they did not absorb what Wang was communicating. In a peak of exasperation, Wang did what only Wang could do...in his world anything was acceptable to encourage the shedding of inhibitions; eccentricity, after all, is one of his specialties. In the name of academic instruction and in furtherance of artistic beauty, Wang pushed the wooden mannequin aside. As it crashed to the floor he stripped himself naked and stood atop a stool, imploring the students to study and draw exactly what was before them! Bear in mind this was 1992 in China.

His instinct for survival and need to self-express no doubt drove Wang to accomplish what he has in life. It also cannot be denied that he has the benefit of natural artistic ability and good genes as well. In addition, he is also highly intelligent and understands the importance of remaining relevant to the here and now. To his credit, he has remained current and successfully avoided being discarded by the art world's ceaseless reinvention of itself. But, as I sat there recording my discussion with Wang, thinking back on his remarks...remembering him as he answered me and all the things he revealed, I came to a different decision about this man and what really drives him...what keeps him on this earth. What forms the foundation of his being? I arrived at one inescapable conclusion...and I know it sounds facile but maybe simplicity is his secret: *Wang has courage…he has more courage in his little finger than most people have in their entire life. He has the audacity to live deliberately with no complaints, embracing all life has to offer…ignoring any obstacle that impedes his passion for living. And that's it really…he has the courage to love life without apology.*

My remarkable time with Wang Deshun, whose name I have come to learn can be roughly translated as "Soft Virtue", was over. But before we said goodbye, I had one more burning question for him. I had to know, after he was gone, for what or how did he want to be remembered? Was it his avant-garde productions on the stages of Beijing? The gift of freedom for expression he taught his students? Maybe the cumulative contributions he made to Chinese modern art? Or perhaps for the barriers he has lowered for the elderly, extending the perceptions of what can be achieved? Each of these is significant and offers a proud, lasting legacy.

"So, Wang, what is your wish?" I asked him pointedly.

Wang smiled broadly and shook his head from side to side denying me each of my suggestions. He glanced at DJ QQ and reached into his pocket. Wang removed a photo and held it up proudly as if he were displaying an official badge: it is a picture of him staring off into the distance with a little girl riding happily on his shoulders. She is laughing and utterly delighted to be carried by him. Despite her innocence, she knows she is safe with her guide…caressing his large ears as she bounces along. And for his part, he has his hands securely on her little legs so that no slip is possible; he is protecting her. In that very instance together their love for each other is clear and I wondered if a photograph has ever revealed such a moment before. It captures perfectly the magic between a father and his child. Wang watched me as I studied the photo. He then said, "Here is your answer. I want to be remembered by my children and grandchildren as a dedicated, loving father...nothing more, nothing less." Ah, I thought to myself, the epitome of courage...he releases all earthy achievements, disengages from every public acknowledgement and yields each material advancement for the everlasting love of his family.

We all sat for a minute quietly. I looked at both DJ QQ and her father absorbing the whole of our conversation. I wanted to say something but DJ QQ jumped ahead of my words and said, "My father is a very spiritual man and worships great nature...he is indeed accomplished but it is his relationships with people that inspire him." With these words, DJ QQ settled the moment nicely.

In full respect of the individual sitting in front of me, I rose and said, "Wang Deshun, you are a complete man, thank you for your story. Wang stood and shook my hand, "I enjoyed our chat...your questions are thoughtful and gave me an opportunity for self-reflection. Not many people ask me these sorts of questions. I wish we had more time to talk but I have to return to my studio...I have a big gig in a month!"

"Understandable...By the way Wang, what is your DJ name?" I asked, full of curiosity right before he left.

Wang turned towards me as he opened the door to the room, the lovely DJ QQ faithfully by his side...he smiled, paused and said with aplomb, "...what else...DJ Old Man!".

DJ QQ escorted her father out of the room and back to the studio. As I walked down the hall I studied the teenagers again, strumming away on guitars with stars in their eyes; singing and laughing out loud, utterly carefree and enjoying their youth to no end. Before I left the studio, I looked back at DJ Old Man and contemplated his life: He is a teenager in spirit...headphones on and dancing away as he blithely mixes his music. Ensconced in his atelier, he is doing what he has always done: using creativity to fearlessly tear down barriers. Only now he bravely sculpts the future by experimenting with the soundtracks of life.

Wang Deshun - Allocation of 9 Essential Relationships

Has	Transition	Has not
Independence and Courage		
Healthy Mind and Spirituality		
Productive Engagement and Community Support		
Happy Heart and Love		
Healthy Body		
Sufficient Wealth		
Strong Family Bonds		
Reliable Friendships		
Self-Respect and Dignity		

Discussion:

Wang Deshun is the paradigm, the *sine qua non* of vitality and robust ageing. He possesses all the Essential Relationships in abundance with nothing even on the cusp of transition. His profile is remarkable. Some might argue that his celebrity status contributed to his success in maintaining Essential Relationships. This is possible and I will acknowledge that it may have played some role but only with regard to his Interpersonal Relationships. His successes with Personal Relationships are witness to his self-knowledge.

Love, Lao Ren Style[7]

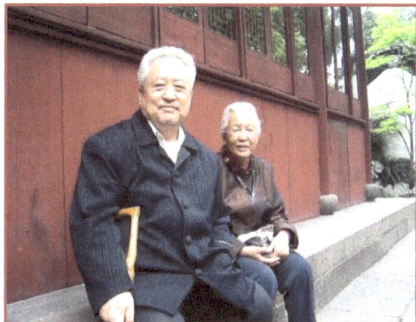

When we are young falling in love is easy. We are emotionally fearless and full of affections. But what happens when we are old and lonely? No longer bold and unafraid, but full of fears, prejudices, insecurities and hesitation which we accumulate over a lifetime? What happens then? This is an improbable story about two senior adults who decide to take a chance with vulnerability and consequently discover the transformative power of love.

The Individuals

<u>Lu Jiabei:</u> From the moment she was able to count, Jiabei was fascinated by symmetry; she yearned to apply her sense of organization to any situation she encountered. To her mind, categorization was harmony, disorder was unpleasant and she was exceedingly good at the process of it all. As class leader throughout primary school she insisted that her peers' form two distinct lines as they queued up for lunch break: one line for girls and one line for boys, shortest to tallest. If there were two classmates of equal

---

[7] Lao Ren: A literal translation means old person in Chinese.

height, then the younger of the two would precede the other in line. She had even provided for the rare instance when two classmates had the same birthdate: the one with the higher score on the most recent exam would prevail. She was prepared for any eventuality. But Jiabei's sense of order was not regimented or harsh. She was never sharp about the imposition of her methods to anyone. Instead she won over cynics to her sense of uniformity through friendly, practical discussion leaving her critic appearing to be a proponent of chaos. In the end, she was simply clever and all her instincts led her to a prosperous business organizing tours and local events.

Jiabei is petite. But size is irrelevant as she is a cerebral powerhouse; a manager at heart, always advancing towards the objective. Today she is 81, a widow and living in *Peace and Serenity*, a senior living development in Wuxi, China. She has lived there since her husband died 7 years ago of an aneurysm. One night as they sat in their living room, he suddenly moaned, called out her name and reached across the sofa for her. As his hand reached her arm and he touched her gently, a final caress and then he collapsed; his head fell into her lap and he was dead. It all happened in five seconds and a lifetime was extinguished in a moment for which she was totally unprepared. She was left feeling betrayed by life as there had been no opportunity to prepare much less say goodbye. Though unfair as she recognized it, dwelling upon this would produce nothing but bitterness, and this was useless to her innate pragmatic self. Six months later she saw no more merit living alone and decided to leave their large house and relocate to *Peace and Serenity*. The decision was easy; Jiabei had no children, no sisters, no brothers and no extended family to consult. Her friends, of which there are many, did indeed support her decision to move. In fact, they were curious about *Peace and Serenity* and promised to visit and inspect for their own purposes as well.

At *Peace and Serenity*, Jiabei was one of the first people to move into the development. That didn't dissuade her from doing what she had always done. Soon after arranging her belongings, she contacted the management and presented a list of items she felt were lacking or could be enhanced. This list was extensive ranging from better organization of the kitchen, improved sales process, additional activities, and so on. From Jiabei's perspective, *Peace and Serenity* was the right place for her...it needed what she had in abundance. The development had potential; it just needed some organizational discipline. It needed her and she knew that. Without a business any longer and with no husband, she desperately needed to belong again.

As the years at *Peace and Serenity* passed, Jiabei became indispensable to the management team. Her instinct for expedited administration was essential and in large part responsible for the facility's curb appeal and rapid occupancy.

Yang Haoming: Haoming is a large man, tall and barrel chested. He is a warm and friendly person, naturally trustworthy and reliable. There is a permanent smile on his face that makes him eminently approachable. For most of his adult life, Haoming was a professor of history at a major university in Shanghai. He is also a good cook, specializing in the delicious dishes from Hunan where his mother was from. From his earliest social encounters as a child, Haoming naturally projected a gravity which drew people to him, although he never purposely sought the spotlight. Today, Haoming is 80 and moved into *Peace and Serenity*, two years ago largely at the prompting, or insistence, of his only child and son, Haishan. Haishan lives in Malaysia and is a busy manager for a major Chinese technology company. Three years ago, Haoming lost his wife after 50 years of marriage. Her death was difficult; she had heart surgery and her recovery was complicated by infection which she never was able to overcome.

For a long time since the heartbreaking moments immediately after her death, Haoming was at a loss. His life was in disarray and their apartment transitioned from a nicely kept two bedroom flat to an unrecognizable mess. He also ate poorly since his wife's passing and has gained a considerable amount of weight. Prior to his move to *Peace and Serenity,* Haoming moped around...aimlessly walking the neighborhood and loitering on corners. At a point nearly 8 months after his wife's death, Haoming became so disconsolate, that two of his friends contacted Haishan and alerted him to his father's odd behavior. Haishan excused himself from his professional obligations and flew to Shanghai the next day.

When Haishan arrived at his father's apartment he was astonished at its condition and immediately knew his father could not continue there. The apartment wasn't just messy; it was disastrous and looked like a burglary had occurred. What surprised Haishan most of all, was that his father had attempted to gather up all of his mother's belongings; there were three suitcases, some full and closed, some partially packed, all containing her clothes and personal effects. Haishan was speechless and tried to discuss the situation with his father...but it was obvious to him that Haoming was deeply troubled by remaining in the apartment. After three days, Haishan concluded his father needed a change and another living arrangement was necessary. For Haoming to remain there might be dangerous. Haishan concluded his father was wasting away and his obvious depression could deepen irreparably.

On the morning of the fourth day of his visit, Haishan's mind was made up. He asked his father to take a small trip with him. They got into a taxi and Haishan gave the driver directions to *Peace and Serenity*. Haoming did not recognize the destination but as taxi drove on, Haishan began to explain where they were going and why. Once he understood, Haoming simply said "no"...he would not consider such a move. But Haishan insisted and told his father that under no circumstances would he permit him to remain in the apartment. Haoming was at a disadvantage in this debate: he could not focus on the argument the way his son could as much of his mind still mourned his wife's passing. Haoming realized as they got closer to *Peace and Serenity* that he would likely lose this quarrel as his son's insistence was berating. Haoming wanted simply to be left alone, be it in his apartment or wherever.

Four months later, Haishan returned to Shanghai and would entertain no further objection to his father's relocation. He had made all the arrangements with *Peace and Serenity* prior to his arrival; after all, the sooner the better in his view: that was the best decision. Haishan further rationalized that Haoming could not come to Malaysia; such a move was out of the question. There were simply too many variables in his life and his father's health was not suitable for the exceedingly hot Malay climate. The morning after Haishan's arrival, he moved his father into an apartment in *Peace and Serenity*. In the afternoon, Haishan signed the paperwork, executed all deposits and paid the final fees. There was no cost to his father...Haishan took care of the entire portion of expense, as a dutiful son should, which exceeded the rent Haoming would receive on his apartment.

The welcoming team helped move Haoming into the one bedroom apartment on the second floor of building D. At four o'clock, Haishan and his father had tea together in the new apartment. Both were silent and didn't speak. An hour later, Haishan needed to take a car back to Pudong airport to catch his return flight to Malaysia. They said goodbye and Haishan promised to return in the fall for the national holiday. In the car ride to Pudong, Haishan fought back his guilt by telling himself his father was safer and better off at *Peace and Serenity*. He was aware that his career was taking an inordinate amount time out of his life...so much so that he was forced to place his father into a senior living facility. Nevertheless,

Haishan reasoned, it was for his father's benefit, even if he lived in Shanghai he would be poorly equipped to care for Haoming. The deed was done; he needed to move on and his father needed to reestablish himself.

The Story in Brief

Introduction: By the end of the week of Haoming's arrival at *Peace and Serenity*, Jiabei was busy preparing welcome messages to the six new residents. She had researched each newcomer and deemed three of them excellent candidates to join a new singing group and she wanted to recruit them quickly. Printing out the invitations, she shut off her computer and headed out to deliver the messages before dinner. On her second delivery, apartment D202, she knocked on the door a few times but there was no answer. Jiabei found this odd as there were no activities going on at that hour and most residents were in their apartments preparing for dinner. She waited for a minute then decided to slip the notice under the door.

As Jiabei turned and began to walk away, the door to D202 opened. She was surprised to see such a large man, and like hers, his hair was fiery white. "Good Afternoon, Sir! I am Lu Jiabei head of the Organizing Committee and I want to welcome you to our new singing club!" Jiabei was polite and energetic.

Haoming for his part was equally surprised to see such a small woman asking him to join a singing group, in fact, it was the first invitation he had received in nearly two years. "I don't sing and just want to be alone." Haoming replied muttering lowly. He began to shut the door when Jiabei chirped again, "Everyone can sing! Just open your heart and let the music out!"

Haoming shut the door and returned to his TV. 'Everyone can sing….open your heart' he mocked Jiabei's words to himself. Then as he sat down on his couch he asked himself out loud 'May I just watch my TV please…?'

Jiabei dismissed Haoming's refusal to join as simply what most newcomers do. In her experience, and according to her records, 75% of new residents usually take 6 months to get used to the environment of *Peace and Serenity*. After which 65% often join in some activity…so she knew there was a good chance to win over Haoming eventually; especially since she had access to his file and knew he was a widower. She knew he would soon seek out new friends.

Haoming took his time settling into *Peace and Serenity*. He was in no rush. Over the next year Haoming gradually grew into the environment and became more at ease with all the residents. His interactions with Jiabei also became more frequent as she often asked him to join one of the many groups she had organized.

The courtship: Two months after his one year anniversary, Haoming was walking from the administrator's office, where he had filed a complaint over poor TV reception, towards the cafeteria for lunch. As he left the office, he decided that instead of the direct path, he would detour and walk through the garden slightly out of the way. As he entered the moon gate, there were a series of stone benches to his left. Haoming's quick eye noticed a lady's pocketbook lying on the second bench. He looked up, scanned the immediate area but saw no one else in the garden…he was alone and reasoned it must have been forgotten by another resident. Instinctively, he picked up the purse and hurried back to the administrator's office and opened the door. A bit out of breathe, Haoming held up the purse so everyone could see it announcing to the three ladies sitting there that he had just found an item in the garden.

Haoming puffed, "Ladies, I found this on my way to the cafeteria...it was on a bench in the garden. There was no one around so I decided to bring it directly to you." The ladies on duty, Jiabei and her two friends were a bit startled.

Quickly understanding the moment for what it was, Jiabei stood up, "Well, what a good deed you have done, Sir! You are the resident of the week I should say!" Jiabei exclaimed. Her two friends looked up at Haoming and nodded in agreement. She approached Haoming and offered to place the bag in the wall safe until it was claimed. The ladies all complimented Haoming and praised him as a hero.

Haoming realized that with this talk about heroes, his action might draw unwanted attention to himself. All he had wanted to do was return the purse to its owner; he had no interest in being called the resident of the week. "No...that is not necessary...please just return the bag to the owner...that is all I wish", Haoming turned quickly and left the administrator's office then headed to the cafeteria. He recognized the woman in the office as that same person who starts all the groups...singing, sewing and Mahjong...he wondered how she had all that energy.

Not more than an hour later, as Haoming was nearly done with his lunch a commotion began at one end of the cafeteria. The squawk of a microphone, some static, then a woman's voice began to speak:

"Ladies and Gentlemen...I have a request. A woman's pocketbook has been discovered by one of our good, honest residents who has returned it to the administration office. If you are missing such an item, please come see me soon!" Jiabei continued..."Our resident does not wish to be identified as he is so humble, but I want everyone to give a round of applause to our secret, honorable policeman!"

Haoming nearly choked on his soup as Jiabei spoke these final words 'honorable policeman'. He gathered himself, said good afternoon to his friends he was sitting with, stood and began to leave the cafeteria as everyone clapped hoping no one would connect him with this Jiabei's words.

As his basic nature was to be outgoing, it was inevitable that Haoming would become more and more immersed in *Peace and Serenity* but he did not want to be singled out. About six months after the episode involving the pocketbook, Jiabei was walking to the Activities Building to attend singing class with some friends when he turned the corner and nearly bumped into a group of ladies.

Haoming apologized for his haste, "Forgive me Ladies, I am careless. I nearly ran into you!"

Jiabei and her friends exclaimed, "Quite alright, Sir, We were not looking where we were going."

"Please allow me…" Haoming reached to open the door to the Activities Building. The ladies lined up, stepped up the single stair and entered the building. It had been raining earlier that morning and as Jiabei took her turn, she miscalculated the height of the stair, suddenly slipped and lost her balance. Haoming was attentive and quickly caught her with his free hand which he swiftly placed behind her back. Jiabei's friends shrieked as they saw her tumble backwards onto the stairs. But Haoming's strength saved her and stopped her fall a split second before her head hit the hard marble step. He clearly had prevented a serious injury.

Jiabei was light; Haoming estimated no more than 35 kilos. But even though she was lean, the dynamic of her fall caught him off balance and he had no choice but to shift his weight, release the door and nimbly move his other hand under her legs to pick her up, thereby regaining his footing. In doing so, Haoming put too much pressure on his left leg and he felt the sudden tear of his thigh muscle. It ripped and the pain shot deep into his back. But he could not release Jiabei or the two of them would have suffered greater injuries; no doubt he would have fallen on her. He summoned all his strength and suppressed the pain. Holding Jiabei in his arms, he asked the ladies to open the door so he could place her on the couch just inside the building. He was concerned that she might faint or possibly have twisted her ankle in the fall. Haoming laid her down gently on the sofa and instructed one of the ladies to get the nurse immediately. Jiabei was dazed...not so much from the slip, but how fast it all had happened. Just how rapidly Haoming had reacted left her breathless.

Jiabei lay there on the sofa and spoke up, "Thank you Haoming. I was very clumsy."

"Are you alright?" Haoming asked..."the nurse will be here any moment. Please stay calm."

"I am fine...luckily no damage" Jiabei replied.

"Let's make sure and have the nurse look at your ankle. That was a nasty twist...you might have hurt yourself badly" Haoming rationalized. He didn't know it but his words were pure caring to Jiabei's ears. This was the first time in years that a man had asked about her well-being much less saved her from an injury. It was at this point that Jiabei realized she was smitten with this gentle giant.

Haoming was kneeling at the sofa's edge speaking to Jiabei when the nurse arrived. As she approached Jiabei, Haoming tried to stand but the pain in his leg and back was so great that he winced horribly and struggled to get upright.

"Haoming!" Jiabei cried..."You are hurt!"

"No...I am fine just an old injury...some stiffness in my back". Haoming regained his balance and excused himself. "You are in good hands now, Jiabei. I am going to leave you to the nurse." Haoming said good bye and limped back to his apartment; the pain was excruciating.

Jiabei's girlfriends watched the whole encounter in awe. They were not sure what to make of this event but they both knew something of material importance had just transpired between their friend and Haoming. Jiabei clearly felt the moment acutely. That evening as she lay in bed with the window open, a soft breeze from the fresh water canals of Wuxi cooled her apartment and she thought about Haoming. This large, handsome man, on two occasions no less, had demonstrated superior character. She tucked her pillow under her head for further support as she fell into reflection. With a deep sigh, she recognized within herself the rise of an emotion that she long ago lost...it was more than a feeling of comfort, more than the sensation of reassurance. For a woman such as Jiabei, whose daily life was founded on order, predictability and equilibrium, Haoming had introduced an element of spontaneity that inspired her to the point of elation. For the first time in years she felt the promise of youth and the sense that the future held excitement. She acknowledged to herself, as she pulled her silk sheet closer, that her feeling for Haoming was a bit scary, but not so much that she felt out of control. She sensed Haoming was trustworthy and that made all the difference. Jiabei closed her eyes and drifted off to sleep as the crisp air refreshed her thoughts and brought her a dream of Haoming and exciting journeys ahead.

For the next two days Haoming could not get out of bed. His leg and back were simply too painful to move for any extended distance. Jiabei was growing increasing concerned not having seen him at all, not in the cafeteria, not in any activity; he was nowhere to be found.

On the afternoon of the third day, Jiabei organized the nurse for a trip to visit Haoming. She felt guilty not having done this earlier but she had held off not wanting to publically appear overly interested. With the nurse in tow, they marched up to Haoming's apartment and knocked on the door...Jiabei announced herself and the nurse's presence in a loud voice so he might hear them even if he were in his bedroom. But Haoming was not in bed, he was in his pajamas watching TV on his couch. When he heard Jiabei's voice he told her and the nurse to enter and was sorry he could not greet them at the door but he was too sore to walk.

Jiabei and the nurse entered immediately and found Haoming drinking tea...looking pained but resting. The nurse immediately began to examine Haoming asking many questions on how and where he had discomfort. After a few minutes, she was satisfied that it was merely a strained muscle and suggested that additional bed rest along with liniment of menthol would speed his recovery. Before she left Haoming's apartment, the nurse insisted he begin to move about in two days' time using a special walker that she would have delivered later in the evening. With her job completed, the nurse said goodnight to both and left.

After the nurse left, Haoming spoke up, "Jiabei, thank you for your concern but I am quickly on the mend. You needn't be too concerned. The nurse herself says I should be ok in a few days."

Jiabei responded flatly, "Haoming, you saved me from a near disaster and hurt yourself in the process. I am indebted to you and must see that you recover...besides, your apartment needs a bit of order." Jiabei was firm as she glanced about the messy apartment with disdain.

Haoming grumbled and Jiabei went about her job setting the apartment in good order. But before she began, she gave Haoming a fresh cup of tea and some fruit from his kitchen. He was now more comfortable and she could get to work tidying up.

For the next week, Jiabei would appear at Haoming's apartment sometimes bringing him breakfast at other times just to visit. Afterwards she would help him stand and learn to maneuver the walker. It was a clumsy device and too much for what Haoming really needed. After some thought, she knew what he required was something smaller and easier to use, which gave Jiabei an idea. The next day, she left *Peace and Serenity* and went to the local market to purchase a stout wooden cane just the right size for Haoming's height and weight. She was very excited about giving it to him and hoped he would like it. Jiabei concocted a plan to gift it to him at tea that afternoon.

Jiabei knocked on Haoming's door and announced herself as she usually did. Haoming responded by asking her to come in...he was in the kitchen cooking and couldn't make to the door so fast with his walker.

Once Haoming opened the door Jiabei inquired, "Are you ready for our walk and some tea in the garden, Haoming?"

Haoming was in a good mood that day as he was beginning to feel stronger, "Yes, I am...and I think I am ready to move away from this darn walker...it is so much trouble."

Jiabei's excitement grew at the prospect of giving Haoming the cane, "Haoming…let's get you downstairs first and see how you are going before we make that move."

Haoming agreed with her and they began the short trek to the garden where Jiabei had a thermos of tea and her gift of a beautiful wooden cane. She carefully hid the cane nearby and planned to present it after a few minutes of friendly discussion.

It was 4pm in early September and unusually dry and cool for that time of year in Wuxi. Jiabei and Haoming both remarked that the garden was very pleasant and next week was an exciting time: Harvest Festival and an auspicious occasion.

After a minute of silence Jiabei spoke, "Haoming…I know I have thanked you for your saving me when I slipped and I don't want to repeat myself but I am grateful…I could have seriously hurt myself and you…you suffered an injury on my behalf."

"Jiabei…please, I am fine now. I was there, I held the door for you and I could not have let you fall. My reflex was automatic. Look at me now…I am nearly fully recovered!" Haoming exclaimed.

Jiabei continued, "Yes…you have recovered nicely. And Haoming…I just want to say that…" Jiabei searched for the words that would precede her giving the gift to Haoming. It was excruciating for her…she needed the right formula of words…her feelings for Haoming hung in the balance.

"Yes…?" Haoming said quizzically.

Jiabei summoned all her courage and then just blurted out, looking directly at Haoming, "Well…I enjoy your company, Haoming…I do. And I want to let you know that." Jiabei stood up quickly and pulled the gift from a stand of bushes next to the bench and presented it to Haoming saying, "Here…this is a gift for you."

Looking up at Jiabei and receiving the cane in both hands, Haoming was bewildered, "What…have you done Jiabei….? I…I am not sure what…" Haoming was speechless.

Jiabei clapped her hands together and chuckled like a school girl, "This is for you Haoming…I bought it for you as I knew you didn't need a walker anymore but a cane might help you from time to time!" Jiabei smiled broadly…she was happy. Haoming passed the cane from one hand to another…it was well polished and had a neatly carved handle. It was obvious to him a great deal of care went into its making.

"Jiabei…thank you…It is a precious and thoughtful gift." At that moment Haoming felt something he had not experienced in years. He was overcome with the feeling of gratitude and compassion for Jiabei. She had been so attentive to him over the past few weeks and now she had gone even further and gifted him a useful cane. As he reviewed his feelings his thoughts took yet another step and he wondered what his life would be like at *Peace and Serenity* without Jiabei. It was a bit confusing to him but abruptly, one thing was clear to him…she was important in his life. Haoming continued to stare at the cane while processing his feelings, trying to understand this new door that was opening in his life.

"Do you like it, Haoming?" Jiabei was concerned with his silence.

Haoming looked back up at Jiabei, "Yes...without a single doubt Jiabei...I was just thinking to myself."

"About what, Haoming...is something wrong?" Jiabei was concerned...she sat down beside him and sympathetically placed her hand on his forearm.

"Jiabei...I am not sure how to say this...I am confused and disoriented...but I would like to make dinner for you tonight...would you accept?" Haoming asked humbly. Seldom had Jiabei heard words more heartfelt and sincere. She could feel his struggle and the courage it took to ask her this question. It was a step on Haoming's part that was prompted by a feeling rather than his rationale; he sensed he was moving through that new open door he recognized a second earlier. Immediately after he asked Jiabei, he realized what he had done and a fear of a possible rejection overcame him.

But Jiabei accepted gratefully, "Oh Haoming...I would love that! Let's go now to the market and buy provisions for our dinner...shall we?" Jiabei was over the moon at this suggestion...she felt young and courted...All her earlier contemplations were now confirmed, she realized that Haoming's presence was exciting for her. For Jiabei, her feelings for Haoming were settled.

Haoming exhaled a lifetime's worth of anxieties hearing Jiabei's words of acceptance. And although Jiabei didn't notice, Haoming's eyes grew red and teary. Instantly, he was full of life and in a way he had not felt since before his wife died. The enchantment of the moment swelled his large heart even larger; invigorating every molecule of his being...he had never felt so alive than at that moment, right then and right there with Jiabei. It was an instant he wished he could keep forever.

<u>Conclusion:</u> For the next year, Jiabei and Haoming spent more and more time together. They vacationed frequently and often prepared dinners in each other's apartments, away from the distracting noise of the cafeteria…and of course the gossip of their neighbors. They took the rumors in stride…as both were aware of their growing affection. By the time I met them, the early days of their courtship were over and it is fair to say that they were a stable couple.

I am in *Peace and Serenity*'s garden with Jiabei and Haoming sitting across from me. They are seated on the same bench where Haoming found the pocketbook. To see them one might think they have been partners for 60 years; holding hands, they smile at each other often and, when I ask a question they turn and gaze into each other's eyes like teenagers…then one of them answers. It is a remarkable sight and hard to fathom just how fortunate they are.

"Haoming and Jiabei…I want to know a lot of things about the two of you," I say, "But most of all I want to know what was the biggest challenge you faced during your courtship?"

Jiabei turns serious for a minute and responds as if she has prepared an outline and beginning to set forth the obstacles. "Well, I will answer for myself and Haoming can tell you his story. For me, I was lonely and although my work here at *Peace and Serenity* is rewarding, I missed male companionship. After I met Haoming, I wanted to learn more about him but I understood he had a hard time before he came here. He needed time to adjust…it wanted to help him but he needed to do it himself. Waiting like that was difficult for me."

"Jiabei, weren't you concerned about entering into a relationship at your age might entail? There is a lot of risk…a lot of things you need to overcome…personal issues?" I pose this direct question to her but I think I know how she will answer.

"No. I was fond of Haoming from the start. He is a very handsome man…tall, smart and kind. I observed his deeds here and there and I was convinced he was a good man." Jiabei responds just as I imagined she might. She tightens her grip on Haoming's large hand and rests her head against his shoulder. Jiabei says one more thing before she is done, "Haoming is a big-hearted man…strong and protective. But he is also the tenderest person I know…so gentle…" Jiabei lets these words drift off and ends her description there.

I think to myself…*'tenderness'*…that is an often overlooked word in a relationship these days. In fact, I seldom hear it. And now Jiabei uses it in a way that expresses both how Haoming treats her and something which she needs. I suppose at their age the software of love: warmth, compassion, sensitivity, tenderness, and of course, understanding, become supreme in a relationship. Then again, I think…of course…these qualities are vital to all relationships; but Jiabei and Haoming, at their age prioritize differently and pay closer attention to these essentials.

"And Haoming," I begin, "Understandably, your experience may have been different. Can you tell me how you came to be so fond of Jiabei?"

Haoming chuckles, "Probably because she is so persistent!" Jiabei smiles at his remark and playfully taps his leg with her hand in an affectionate motion. I recognize that small gesture on Jiabei's part, it underscores how comfortable they have become with one another.

"Yes, she is…I can see that," I say, "But, Haoming…tell me about the difficult times…can you?"

Haoming begins immediately, "My son, Haishan was firmly against any communication with Jiabei. I tried to ask him why he felt so strongly about this but his argument was mostly in support of his own feelings and not mine. He accused her of all sorts of terrible things…even conspiring to take my old apartment from me. Haishan even spoke to the manager of *Peace and Serenity*…He felt she was a menace and would lead to trouble for me. But, there was another problem also. And I know this only now because I took a risk and was lucky. But, I was afraid…afraid of a lot of things. Mostly, I was fearful about liking Jiabei and what that might mean for me. I never thought I could be so comfortable again in my life. But Jiabei made it safe for me to express how I felt." Haoming, at 80 years old, shows extraordinary self-awareness. His words are simple but they provide a complete picture of his journey.

"What does Haishan say now?" I wonder out loud to Haoming.

Haoming shrugs his shoulders, "Regrettably, he hasn't spoken to me in 5 months since I told him that Jiabei was now my girlfriend. I tried to explain to him that this is my life and I need to be happy."

"Wow…" I am amazed at the turn of events I am hearing. It appears to be a reversal of roles between parent and child. I hope that Haishan comes around and can appreciate what, in a very real way, he enabled for his father.

Haoming continues, "Haishan was angry and said I did not show him any gratitude for saving me from my squalid existence at my old apartment. But I told him, the contrary was true: I was indeed very grateful because if it was not for him, I would not have met Jiabei…He was very angry at that remark."

"So, here we are…Haoming and Jiabei in love…and happy at *Peace and Serenity*. What happens next?" I ask them both.

Jiabei, who had been silent for much of the last few minutes resting her head on Haoming's large frame, perks up at my question.

"First, thing is that we are going to consolidate our apartments! That is the most economical decision now. We can save quite a lot of money. Second, we are planning a small vacation to Hainan. This will give us a nice break from *Peace and Serenity*" Jiabei is giddy at these prospects.

"Congratulations!" I said. I am a bit surprised with this last piece of information. I continue, "I am curious, what do all your friends say to you here at *Peace and Serenity*?"

Jiabei jumps at this answer, "Oh they tease us and call us kids…but I think it is all in good fun. Perhaps they envy us."

I nod in agreement. Of this I am certain…envy…possibly jealousy and maybe even some condescension. I then ask, "And the management…have they commented at all?"

Jiabei responds again, "I spoke with them early on when they inquired after rumors that had been swirling at *Peace and Serenity*…I reminded them of our independence. They are no longer concerned." I can imagine this conversation…Jiabei was no doubt her practical self…crafting a forceful argument and trapping management in a position where they found themselves in a predicament: arguing against the happiness of their residents. It seems as if Jiabei, as only she could, effectively silenced this matter.

Haoming and Jiabei announce that they are late for their calligraphy class and must get going. We stand and say goodbye, they turn and walk on; Haoming using his cane with one hand, his other arm warmly around Jiabei's shoulders. In turn she wraps her arm around his waist. They disappear around the corner and back into their private lives, supporting each other and together, leaning into life.

For my part, I sit back down and begin to put all the pieces of this inspiring story together. I am not sure if it is complicated or simple; maybe I am just trying to make it complicated. But I am left with two irrefutable facts: first, Jiabei and Haoming are clearly in love, however unlikely that might be, second, in order to get to where they are now, they needed to defeat a life time's worth of protective experience in order to prevail over their fears and reveal to each other their vulnerabilities...which no doubt was difficult. Each of them, in their quiet moments, struggled to understand their attraction to one another and its implications. I am certain from time to time they independently reasoned that either the safety of their apartment or being cloistered away with friends might be more wise, avoiding the risk of hurt.

Exactly how Haoming and Jiabei's relationship happened remains a mystery. But perhaps early on they recognized that each one offered the other something that is at the heart of what the other needed. Indeed there is proportionality, a fit to them that is rare. Maybe it just felt so good to be together that there was no denying it...or maybe they never really spoke outwardly about it and it just happened. There are a lot of maybe's here...it is difficult to analyze the chemistry of Jiabei and Haoming. What is important is that their lives have undergone rejuvenation.

Before we parted I asked them one last question which I hoped might reveal more about what they think of themselves. I asked them whether, had they had met 60 years ago, would they have fallen in love?...Is their attraction to each other intrinsic?...Is it destiny?...Or is it more related to their environment and their needs today? Their answer is surprising...and almost in unison they respond that their love for each other is all about today, where they are presently and what each needs now. In fact, I believe they feel that their histories are irrelevant. There is no fantasy here, no pretense of long lost soulmates, they are mature adults and both firmly rooted in reality, which is refreshing. For them being together is spontaneous and to be so unconstrained at their age is a miraculous and wonderful thing.

I sit in the garden for another minute watching other seniors walk around...some alone, some in groups and a few couples; none of whom seem as alive as do Haoming and Jiabei. The thought occurs to me that what I have listened to is a transcendental chronicle on the enduring and regenerative nature of love that proves how an affectionate human bond, fortified with compassion, is a force for positive transformation. Indeed, finding a devoted relationship at their age has no equivalent...and nothing...no spa treatment, no tai chi class, no yoga session, no enzyme or stem cell therapy could be more curative than Love, Lao Ren Style.

Lu Jiabei and Yang Haoming - Allocation of 9 Essential Relationships

Jiabei

Has	Positive Transition ←	Has not
Self-Respect and Dignity	Happy Heart and Love	Strong Family Bonds
Healthy Mind and Spirituality		
Independence and Courage		
Productive Engagement and Community Support		
Healthy Body		
Reliable Friendships		
Sufficient Wealth		

Haoming

Has	Positive Transition ←	Has not
Self-Respect and Dignity	Happy Heart and Love	Strong Family Bonds
Healthy Mind and Spirituality	Independence and Courage	
Sufficient Wealth	Productive Engagement and Community Support	
Healthy Body	Reliable Friendships	

Discussion:

Jiabei: Jiabei is a remarkable woman. She has navigated her life with enormous thought and care. Of all the interviews she is one of only three profiles with so many retained Essential Relationships, possessing seven of the 9 Essential Relationships with one in Positive Transition.

Haoming: Haoming is a sweet man and, from an Essential Relationship point of view, the true beneficiary of the union between him and Jiabei. Prior to his meeting Jiabei, his future looked bleak. He had lost his wife and only possessed three Essential Relationships. But having met Jiabei, he has four Essential Relationships in Positive Transition; his profile is unique in this regard and speaks to the story's fundamental premise that love is a positive force multiplier and has the power to revitalize.

There are only two couples in this book: Jiabei - Haoming and Jun – Shishang. The two couples present a shocking study in contrasts.

Welcome Home, Mr. Shen

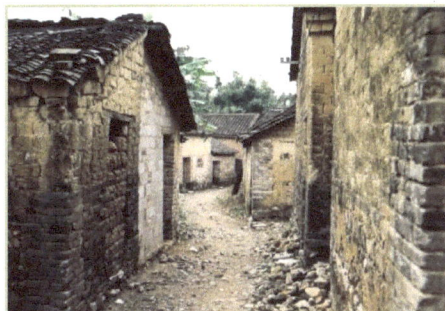

Shen Dihan was born in 1925 in a small village near Bo Zhou, a rural city in northeastern Anhui Province. Bo Zhou is known as the TCM capital of China and has a distinct history stemming back to the days of the Eastern Han Dynasty. Shen Dihan has a number of terminal health conditions: He has advanced renal disease and is without frequent hemodialysis which has resulted in complicated uremia. To make matters worse, eight months ago Shen Dihan suffered a stroke which left him speechless. The following is an account of the last day of his life.

[I can feel the tall wheat rub up against my thighs. The wheat's spikelets are sharp and prick my legs as I run through the field. Yesterday was my 6th birthday and I am now a big boy and can go to the catacombs without my brother...besides I know the passages better than him. I can see Zhang Yu in the distance waiting for me at the entrance to the underground tunnels. She is my best playmate and we often spend the whole day together while our parents work in the fields. Zhang Yu now waves at me, begging me to run faster. I can see she is carrying a small bag...possibly with a snack and

candle! The tunnels are dark. It is September and hot in the field but the catacombs are refreshing; they are cool and damp.]

I open my eyes. I am aware of three things: first, I am dreaming; second, I am in great pain; third, the doctors are moving about me. Two nurse aides gather about and shift my body to one side in a futile effort to treat my pressure ulcers. As they turn me the hurting is too much to bear…

["Hurry Shen Dihan…Your brother is coming!" Zhang Yu beckons to me.

"I am coming…enter the tunnel now!" I cry back.

I approach the entrance to the first catacomb. I turn quickly and see my brother in full stride only 300 meters away. I duck under the stone headwall and into the tunnel. Zhang Yu is waiting for me and I take her hand and we pass by the main passageway and chose the smaller path just beyond. I know of a secret shaft where we can hide until brother passes and we are safe. I raise my finger to my mouth and motion for Zhang Yu to be silent. The shaft-way ahead is small but we can fit…brother is too big. Together we enter the small space…the walls are cold. I dare not light the candle as brother would see the light so I must feel my way into the space and find a comfortable area to lie until it is safe to leave. I continue to hold Zhang Yu's hand and calm her…she is frightened and the cold stone makes her shiver. I turn my head and whisper into her ear, "Brother will be here in only a few minutes…he does not know these passages like we do and he has no candle. He will leave soon…stay calm Zhang Yu."

Zhang Yu squeezes my hand acknowledging my advice. Her little hand fits nicely in mine. We are close and I feel warm and responsible when we are together. She is kind and says supportive words to me.]

The doctors are above me once again. The lights above are blinding and they are poking at me with instruments; attacking me with technological interventions, robbing me of peace and humanity. I feel like a living experiment…merely a body on which they practice. They have no knowledge of my extreme discomfort. I want only to return to the catacombs and Zhang Yu…

[*"Zhang Yu…we can go now. Brother has passed and grown tired of looking for us. Come with me now," I say, reporting the conditions to my beloved playmate and she agrees. I help her shuffle between the massive stone columns and we step down back onto the tunnel's dirt floor.*

"Shen Dihan, where shall we go now?" Zhang Yu asks me out loud.

"Let's proceed down the main corridor and into the large room. There is a side passage that leads to our eating room. We can play castle there for a while," I propose to Zhang Yu. Playing castle is our most fun game. We imagine I am an emperor and she my queen: these catacombs are our castle and it protects us from the invaders. I know today we will have hours of imaginative fun. She is my best friend and I hope we never part.]

The machine is now inside me again. It removes my blood and pumps it back into me. It is a monster and has no respect for me. It is eating me. It will not cure me. How can I defeat this fiend? I just want to be left to my dream. I want to return to Zhang Yu and the tunnels. I can hear the doctors speak again about me and my status. I understand I am to be moved. Some people have been allowed to take me away. I am to be removed from the hospital! I want to disconnect the machine. Please allow me to sleep. I want the dignity with which I was endowed at birth. Please give me respect and let me go…

[*"Queen! Can we eat lunch now? I ask Zhang Yu.*

"Yes, my Emperor. I have a nice cake for us!" Zhang Yu unfolds the small cloth sack and removes a cake she took from home. It is tiny and broken but it is a good snack.

"After we eat lunch I will clean our castle Emperor," Zhang Yu reports on her duties for the game to continue. She is an eager playmate and makes our game truly fun.

"Good idea, Queen. I will secure the doors and lock the gates so we are protected from the invaders," I reassure Zhang Yu as to my duty. We are equal partners in this fantasy; each of us promotes the other and wants the game to succeed.

"Please Shen Dihan, protect us from them? You must fight the invader. They are relentless!" Zhang Yu pleads with her little mouth full of cake.

"Always my Queen...I will not let them harm us," I take my last bite of cake and want to impress Zhang Yu with my diligence. I stand and pretend I am locking the gates. Zhang Yu watches me affectionately. I think to myself, 'I will defeat these terrible invaders no matter what.']

Oh...Pain! The orderlies are lifting me from my bed and taking me away. But at least the monstrous machine is gone; I have overcome this horrible intruder. There is a long discussion about me and warnings given by the doctors. I am in a car now we are traveling...

["Zhang Yu, your Emperor is tired from so much work. I will rest now." I say as I know what happens in the next stage of our castle game. I now lie down on the large stone.

"Emperor, please rest and don't get sick." Zhang Yu says as she kneels down by my side. She holds my hand and is worried about my health.

"Be strong for me Zhang Yu. Your emperor has defeated the invader but now I simply need rest to for my next challenge," I beg her to allow me some reprieve.]

I now recognize my surroundings. I am home. People around me are my old friends and they welcome me home. They have saved me from the hospital and brought me to my castle. No more machines, no more doctors. My beloved Zhang Yu is next to me. She is old but always beautiful. She kneels and holds my hand. She is crying but I cannot hear her words. She leans over to embrace me. I close my eyes, no longer in pain. I feel human again. I am in my home and at peace. I now have my pride back and I am prepared for my next challenge...

[*"Zhang Yu...everything is okay. I just need some sleep. The invaders are gone forever," I say trying to comfort her. I am ready to go now.*

"My Emperor..." Zhang Yu begs with tears streaming down her cheeks, "I will help you in your next challenge; I will be by your side forever."

"Zhang Yu, we are safe. We are together and nothing can harm us. It is time to rest." I speak these words as Zhang Yu reaches over me and embraces me warmly. My eyes close and I no longer feel the cold stone, just the warmth of Zhang Yu holding me.]

Shen Dihan - Allocation of 9 Essential Relationships

<u>Has</u>	<u>Positive Transition</u> ←	<u>Has not</u>
Reliable Friendships	Self-Respect and Dignity	Independence and Courage
		Healthy Mind and Spirituality
		Productive Engagement and Community Support
		Happy Heart and Love
		Healthy Body
		Sufficient Wealth
		Strong Family Bonds

Discussion:

Shen Dihan was terminally ill. In his final days, he only wanted pain relief and to die at home with dignity among people he loved and who loved him. The ultimate act of caring was when his friends removed him from the hospital and returned him to his home to be among his people as he passed away.

In Shen Dihan's particular case, the acquisition of an Essential Relationship does not extend his life, but it does make him happier in the end.

Appendix

Farewell my Migrant Health Care Worker

(Reprint from *"Enter the Ageing Dragon"* 2013)

告 别 了 流 动 护 理 工 时 代

"A smile ushers in the Spring and a tear does darken all the world", Master Yuan in
Farewell my Concubine

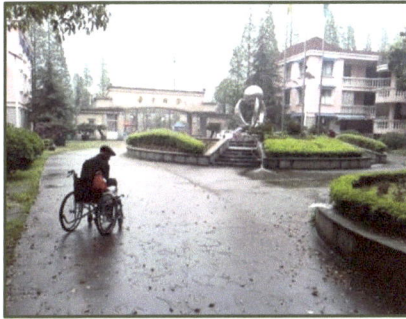

同 志 好! What follows below is a slightly edited transcript of an interview with a young woman named "Jiang" (alias) which occurred in Beijing, Chaoyang District at a Starbucks coffee shop on December 1, 2011. All edits are primarily due to issues of translation, my imperfect "on the run" typing effort and a very uncomfortable seat at Starbucks. Otherwise, her responses are reported below in as true a form as possible. The purpose of the interview is to shed light on the single most critical issue within the burgeoning geriatric care industry in China: namely, the absolute dearth of properly trained human resources and consequently the use of inadequately trained personnel to administer care to the elderly Chinese. A read through the interview illuminates other social concerns, and while I am sympathetic to these, my focus here is senior care.

Jiang is a young lady of 36 years who is a migrant health care worker in Beijing. She is perfectly average for her social cohort in nearly every respect: neither pretty nor ugly, simply dressed, with serious tooth decay and a limited world view. She is a contract employee at a state run nursing facility and has no professional education in nursing other than what she has learned over the past few years. Jiang, and many of the people with whom she works are known as "Bao Mu", or migrant workers. Being Bao Mu carries a stigma and it is not a pleasant one; they are viewed as wholly inferior, as a lower caste, dirty and unworthy. Bao Mu are usually ethnic minorities and they have largely been disenfranchised from the Chinese economic miracle. In reality, I found in Jiang bucolic charm and a meek honesty which set her in sharp contradiction to her current urban existence; indeed, to her, life in Beijing could not be more uncomfortably foreign.

As we moved through the discussion, Jiang became more relaxed and began to open up. I did not intend to enter the realm of her private life but as the interview progressed, it became obvious that her past has had profound influence on her current situation. Some of her answers are startling and painful; they paint a vivid picture of not only her job but of her life as well. Lastly, you will notice that the conversation is occasionally peppered with anecdotal comments, either before or after a question, in << >> brackets. I added these notes after a final proof read as I found a simple rote reproduction of the interview resulted in a hollowness which failed to sufficiently convey the emotional environment.

Jiang arrived at Starbucks prior to the translator and me. She was sitting at a small table in the back of the room waiting patiently with her coat and gloves on, giving a guarded impression that she considered us a potential no-show. As we approached the table she stood, smiled and said hello. After a brief introduction by the translator and some explanation, I began the interview:

Bromme 柯博明: Hello, Jiang.

Jiang: Hello Sir.

Bromme 柯博明: My name is 柯博明 and I have a business here in China. I help Chinese businesses build private nursing homes and senior living facilities. I have explained to you that I want to ask you a number of questions about the work you do, how you came to do it, what you think about it and generally about what you want to do in the future. Is this ok? You understand?

Jiang: Yes Sir.

Bromme 柯博明: Also, I am asking you these questions because I intend to publish your answers on a website I own and eventually include them in a book. You will remain anonymous, but your responses will be reproduced, after translation and small edits, in their entirety. This is ok for you?

Jiang: Yes Sir.

<<Jiang nods in approval>>

Bromme 柯博明: Ok, let's get started. Where were you born and where did you grow up?

Jiang: I was born in Bishan...I grew up there too; my entire life.

<<Bishan is a rural town near Chongqing. Jiang, obedient and dutiful, asks if she can take her coat off.>>

Bromme 柯博明: How old are you?

Jiang: 36

<<She honestly looked much, much older...I was guessing 45>>

Bromme 柯博明: How many years of education do you have? And what have you studied?

Jiang: I studied the basic curriculum.

<<This means that Jiang spent nine years in school>>

Bromme 柯博明: Jiang, I understand that you work in a nursing home, how long have you worked there?

Jiang: About three years...

Bromme 柯博明: What do you like most about it?

Jiang: The money, but I do not get paid much.

Bromme 柯博明: How much are you paid?

<<*Glancing between the translator and me, Jiang was not eager to discuss her salary and I think she found this a little intrusive. There was some conversation between them about my question between the time I asked it and her final response. It was awkward for her and, I sensed a little painful. But I believe she was truthful.*>>

Jiang: They pay me 1,500 RmB per month. I also get a bed and some food.

<<*This equates to roughly USD235 plus the food and bed.*>>

Bromme 柯博明: What do you like least about it?

Jiang: I do not like taking care of old people; I am a young person. The old people yell at me and sometimes try and hit me when I have to touch them.

Bromme 柯博明: Do you get hit a lot? Why do you have to touch them? What do you mean?

Jiang: Sometimes I get hit but often they miss me because they are slow. The nurses tell me I have to clean them when they shit in the bed. Or sometimes I have to help them go to the bathroom by inserting my finger into their anus. Also, sometimes the families blame us when the old people die.

<<*Jiang tried to release this bit of information as if she were sorting laundry, but she could not contain the anguish; it was embarrassing for her.*>>

Bromme 柯博明: Does anyone else hit you? Have the nurses every hit you? The boss?

Jiang: No. My father used to hit me but not the nurses.

<<I choked on my breath. Obviously, this was unexpected and the result of a miscue in translation. It made both the translator and me a little uncomfortable, and I decided to ignore it for the time being. After a breath, I continued.>>

Bromme 柯博明: How did you find your job here at the nursing home?

Jiang: My friends told me.

Bromme 柯博明: How did they find this job?

Jiang: I don't know.

Bromme 柯博明: What did you do before you worked at the nursing home?

Jiang: I was a food worker. I prepared food in a factory.

<<Her answers here were robotic and truly conveyed that she was disconnected to her job; it was merely a means to an end>>

Bromme 柯博明: Jiang, when you left the factory (Where was the factory?) and came here to Beijing to work at the nursing home, what training did they give you?

Jiang: I worked in Wenzhou. When I was contracted, the nurses told me what to do and after a few weeks I was able to do most of the work alone.

<<Wenzhou is located on the coast of China, not far south of Shanghai. Wenzhou is the crucible of Chinese entrepreneurship>>

Bromme 柯博明: And today, do you work unsupervised?

Jiang: Yes, most of the day.

Bromme 柯博明: Other than clean the patients, what else are your duties?

Jiang: I feed them, give them medicine, help wash them, help them exercise if they want.

Bromme 柯博明: Jiang, how long do you think you will work at the nursing home? Do you have other plans? What would you like to do with your life after the nursing home?

<<This question was either puzzling to Jiang or the translation was off. It took a few iterations to get it on target>>

Jiang: I have to work here because I need the money. Someday I might find another job but I don't know. I would like not to work here, but I don't know where to go. I would like to have a shop and sell things.

Bromme 柯博明: What type of things would you like to sell?

Jiang: All sorts of things, cute little knickknacks, dolls, sweets!

<<Jiang turned into a little girl describing this. She was almost excited and literally disappeared into another world for a moment>>

Bromme 柯博明: So, Jiang, if I understand you correctly, you work at the nursing home for no other reason than you need the money? Right? You essentially hate the job, nothing about it interests you. In fact, caring for the old people disgusts you...they even hit you sometimes, right?

Jiang: Yes Sir.

Bromme 柯博明: Do you think you are good at your job? Are you proud to be a health care worker?

Jiang: Today I know my job and I do it, but I do not like it. I am not proud of being a health care worker...it is a low job.

<<The idea of being proud of her job was novel, but once she understood the question, she responded with little hesitation>>

Bromme 柯博明: Do you think being a health care worker is an important job?

Jiang: It is not an important job, if it were I would be paid more money.

<<Jiang's logic was unassailable and her honesty was simple. I was beginning to sense that this idea of mine, that is to interview a migrant health care worker, needed something more. So I decided on a different track>>

Bromme 柯博明: I want to ask you some questions not related to your job at the nursing home, ok?

Jiang: Yes.

Bromme 柯博明: Did you have a happy childhood and are your parents still alive?

<<I felt this was a reasonable subject to explore given her prior admission about her father>>

Jiang: My parents are alive. We are a very poor family. And when I was little my parents had to split up and work in different cities. I had to go and live with my relatives for a long time. One day my father came to get me and take me home. But he would beat me all day and tell me to call my mother and beg her to come home. I had a very bad relationship with my father.

<<Jiang opened up here in a way that I doubt she has in quite some time. She was almost eager to say these things. Her answer above is an abridged version of her entire response>>

Bromme 柯博明: If you could buy anything what would it be?

Jiang: A nice house for my mother and a shop for me!

<<Jiang smiled broadly. She missed her mother enormously>>

Bromme 柯博明: Jiang, I have only a few more questions. When your mother is old and frail will you take care of her? Or would you consider a nursing home for her?

Jiang: Yes, I will care for her.

<<Jiang oozed empathy>>

Bromme 柯博明: But you will have to work, right? How will you take care of her and work at the same time?

Jiang: I don't know.

<<And again, Jiang's honesty was never more apparent than in this answer. She paused for a while before answering, looked down at the floor hopelessly and responded without looking up. I think that this may have been the first time she ever considered the difficult situation of either caring for the mother she loves more than anything or supporting herself. I don't want to read too much into her answer but I suspect that she began to rethink her plight at this moment. Her answer in a way almost made me feel guilty about presenting her with this dilemma>>

Bromme 柯博明: Jiang, do you have any questions for me?

Jiang: Sir, why do you want to work in nursing homes?

<<Clever girl, I thought>>

Bromme 柯博明: I don't really work in them. I help people build them and operate them.

<<Jiang waited for the translation. It didn't appear that my response really answered her question>>

Bromme 柯博明: Thank you, Jiang. I have enjoyed speaking with you.

Jiang: Yes Sir. Did I do a good job?

Bromme 柯博明: Yes, Jiang. You did a great job.

<<Jiang rose from the table and put her jacket back on. She thanked the translator, smiled and began to walk out, when I asked her one last question>>

Bromme 柯博明: Oh, ah…Jiang..?

Jiang: Yes Sir?

<<Jiang pauses and turns to look at me…she smiles broadly>>

Bromme 柯博明: Have you ever seen the Chinese movie *Farewell My Concubine*?

Jiang: Oh, no Sir, I don't know what that is. Anyway movies are too expensive. Goodbye!

Bromme 柯博明: Goodbye, Jiang.

<<Jiang turned and walked towards the exit. For all the weight she carried on her small shoulders, she had a carefree bounce in her step as she slid through the glass doors and waved one last time.>>

In my two hours with her, I found Jiang to be much like Chen Dieyi in the film *Farewell my Concubine.* Not on a superficial level, but in terms of how tortured she must be; caught in the middle of a miserable triangle with the angles of her life defined by a father who beat her as a child, the necessity of holding down a job she despises and a mother to whom she is fully devoted and loves dearly but cannot live with for financial reasons. Making this mosaic more complex, Jiang knows that she, like millions of other poor and middle income Chinese, face a dreadful dilemma of ultimately having to care for their parents and lose a job or keep the job and turn their parents over to a nursing home. This dynamic is one reason for the decline of traditional filial piety in China and its evolution into something more modern that will make facility living an acceptable option.

Update: Last week I found myself in the vicinity of the nursing home where Jiang works. I stopped by to say hello and thank her again for her time. The manager of the facility seemed frustrated when I inquired about her; he told me she had quit her job three days ago and did not know where she went.

She just left he explained, raising his hands in exasperation, "Like all the Bao Mu, appear from nowhere and disappear into nowhere".

I turned and walked out of the nursing home, leaving behind the caustic tang of bleach and sour reek of dirty clothes. The cold air bit into my nose and cleared my lungs as I stepped outside. I walked down the street and thought about what the manager said regarding Bao Mu disappearing into nowhere. As I hailed a cab I looked back at the nursing home and imagined Jiang, an apparition with suitcase in hand, furtively leaving her job, escaping under the cover of a foggy dawn.

Full of ephemeral sympathy for Jiang, I thought to myself as I got into the cab and closed the door, "Indeed...'disappearing into nowhere' has there ever been a more poignant, unknown destination?"

Personal and Interpersonal Relationship Data

Below are a series of tables which tabulate the allocations of the 9 Essential Relationships.

Have	Xiuyu	Jun	Shishang	Xiaohong	Mrs Jiang	Su Xiu	Wang Deshun	Jiabei	Haoming	Mr. Shen	Line totals	Column Totals
Personal Relationship												
Healthy Mind		1	1	1	1	1	1	1	1		8	
Healthy Body	1		1				1	1	1		5	
Happy Heart		1				1	1				3	
Independence					1	1	1	1			4	
Sufficient wealth							1	1	1	1	4	
Self respect		1		1		1	1	1	1		6	30
Interpersonal Relationship												
Strong family bonds						1	1				2	
Reliable friendships				1		1	1	1		1	5	
Productivity				1		1	1	1			4	11

<u>Observations with regard to Have and Have not allocations:</u> From a **Have** perspective, allocations for Personal Relationships dominated the Profiles compared with Interpersonal Relationships. 9 out of 10 profiles possessed Personal Relationships with the average being 5. Of the 60 potential allocations for Personal Relationships (6 PR multiplied by 10 Profiles) 50% (normalization: 30 allocations divided by 60 potential allocations) possessed a Personal Relationship whereas only 36% (normalization: 11 allocations divided by 30 potential allocations) possessed an Interpersonal relationship. The most commonly **Have** Personal Relationship is a Healthy Mind followed by equal allocations of Healthy Body and Self-Respect.

Have not	Xiuyu	Jun	Shishang	Xiaohong	Mrs Jiang	Su xiu	Wang Deshun	Jiabei	Haoming	Mr. Shen	Line totals	Column Totals
Personal Relationship												
Healthy Mind	1									1	2	
Healthy Body				1	1					1	3	
Happy Heart	1			1						1	3	
Independence	1		1	1						1	4	
Sufficient wealth	1	1	1	1	1					1	6	
Self respect											0	18
Interpersonal Relationship												
Strong family bonds	1	1	1	1	1			1	1	1	8	
Reliable friendships	1	1	1		1						4	
Productivity	1	1	1		1					1	5	17

In contrast, the **Have not** allocations for Personal and Interpersonal relationships exhibit different correlation than do the **Have** allocations. On a normalized basis, Profiles with **Have not** allocations of Interpersonal Relationships (49%) are nearly equal when compared with the **Have not** Personal Relationships (51%). It would appear that when the elderly lack Essential Relationships, they lack Personal Relationships and Interpersonal Relationships in nearly the same proportion.

Assessment: No conclusions can be drawn from this data but potential links and correlations might be inferred. For example, the appearance that

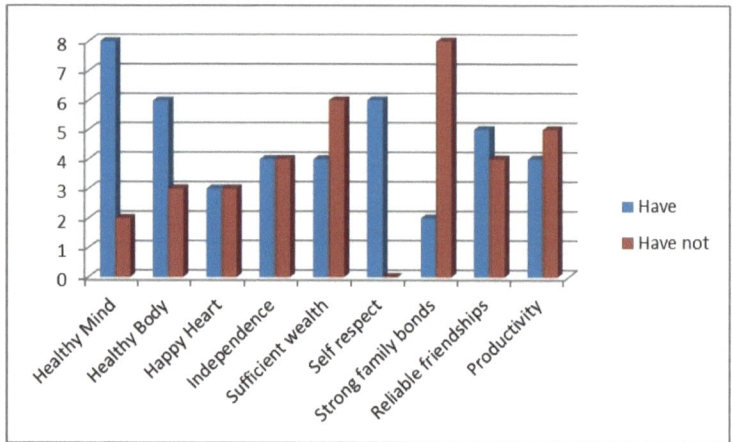

Personal Relationships seem to have a dominate position over Interpersonal Relationships is certainly an area that is deserving of additional study. Further, the Essential Relationships of Healthy Mind, Healthy Body and Self-Respect all command the greatest **Have** allocations while Strong Family Bonds accounts for the largest **Have not** allocation. The least common **Have** allocation for Personal Relationship is a Happy Heart. One can imagine that there are underlying dynamics that might explain these findings. Further study is clearly warranted.

Neg TRANSITION	Xiuyu	Jun	Shishang	Xiaohong	Mrs Jiang	Su xiu	Wang Deshun	Jiabei	Haoming	Mr. Shen	Line totals	Column Totals
Personal Relationship												
Healthy Mind											0	
Healthy Body		1				1					2	
Happy Heart			1								1	
Independence		1									1	
Sufficient wealth											0	
Self respect	1		1								2	6
Interpersonal Relationship												
Strong family bonds											0	
Reliable friendships											0	
Productivity											0	0

<u>Observations with regard to Negative and Positive Transitions:</u> There are 4 profiles that have **Negative Transitions**: Xiuyu, Jun, Shishang and Su Xiu. 75% of them have died: Xiuyu, Jun and Shishang. The three that died had an average of only 2 Personal Relationships. There is yet another point of commonality among these three profiles that merits comment: all three

Pos TRANSITION	Xiuyu	Jun	Shishang	Xiaohong	Mrs Jiang	Su xiu	Wang Deshun	Jiabei	Haoming	Mr. Shen	Line totals	Column Totals
Personal Relationship												
Healthy Mind											0	
Healthy Body											0	
Happy Heart					1			1	1		3	
Independence									1		1	
Sufficient wealth											0	
Self respect					1					1	2	6
Interpersonal Relationship												
Strong family bonds											0	
Reliable friendships									1		1	
Productivity									1		1	2

deceased profiles share a complete lack of Interpersonal Relationships. Regarding Su Xiu, she is a unique profile and will no doubt survive her **Negative Transition** as she has 8 Personal Relationships.

Remarks on the 4 Profiles in **Positive Transition** is best illustrated in the narrative form of their stories. However, of the 4 profiles with **Positive Transition** only Mr. Shen has passed, which, curiously, is the opposite finding from the **Negative Transition** profiles. This would seem to support the fundamental premise of the Social Engagement Theory that **Positive Transitions** promote successful living.

Timeline

Timeline of Chinese History with Life Span of Profiles

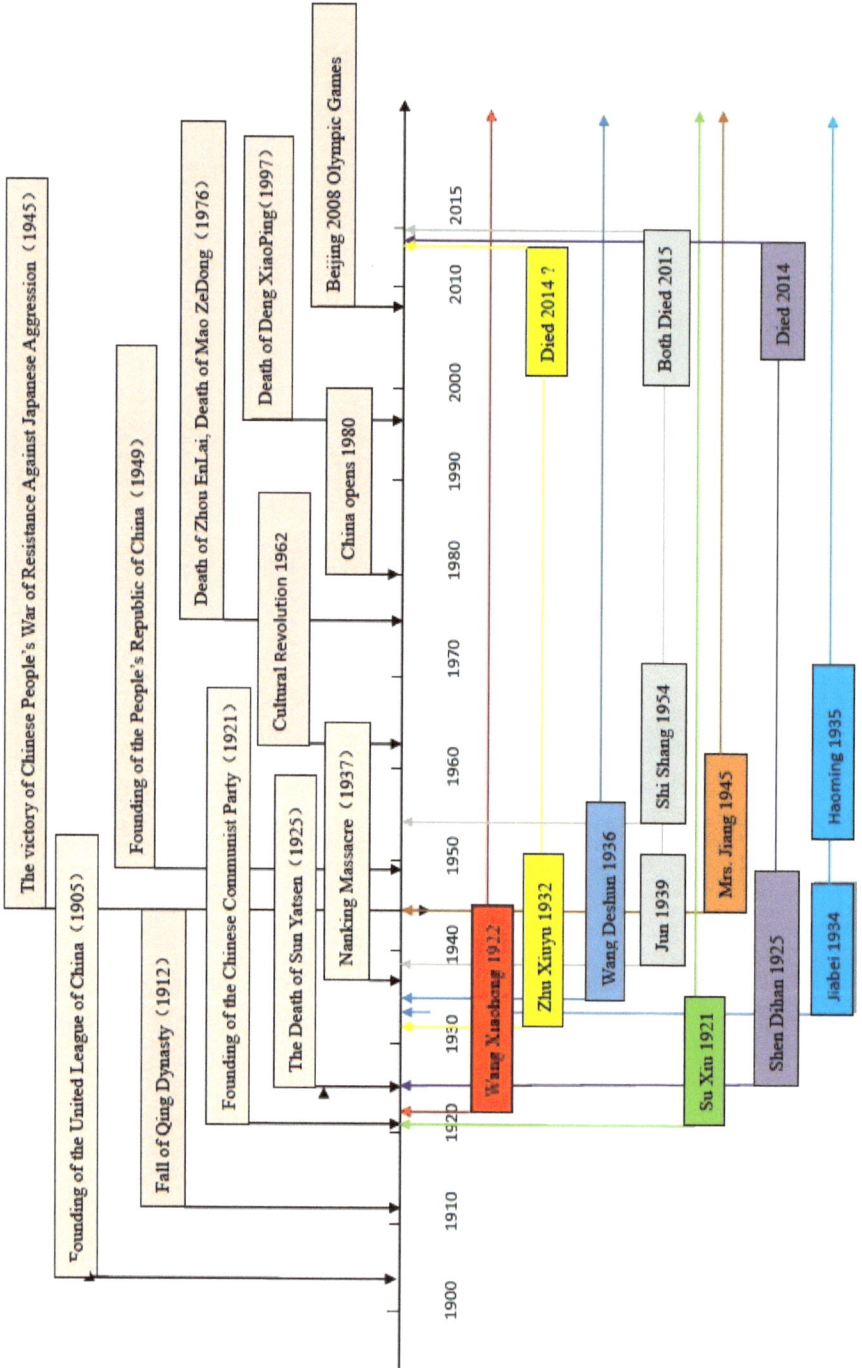

Founding of the United League of China（1905）

The victory of Chinese People's War of Resistance Against Japanese Aggression（1945）

Founding of the People's Republic of China（1949）

Death of Zhou EnLai, Death of Mao ZeDong（1976）

Death of Deng XiaoPing（1997）

Beijing 2008 Olympic Games

Fall of Qing Dynasty（1912）

Founding of the Chinese Communist Party（1921）

Cultural Revolution 1962

China opens 1980

The Death of Sun Yatsen（1925）

Nanking Massacre（1937）

Wang Xiaodong 1922

Zhu Xinyu 1932

Wang Deshun 1936

Jun 1939

Mrs. Jiang 1945

Haoming 1935

Shi Shang 1954

Died 2014 ?

Both Died 2015

Died 2014

Su Xin 1921

Shen Dihan 1925

Jiabei 1934

1900　1910　1920　1930　1940　1950　1960　1970　1980　1990　2000　2010　2015

Support for Social Engagement Theory for Chinese Ageing

"A Continuity Theory of Normal Aging"

Robert C. Atchley, PhD
 Author Affiliations
1Miami University Oxford, Ohio 45056

Abstract:

Continuity Theory holds that, in making adaptive choices, middle-aged and older adults attempt to preserve and maintain existing internal and external structures; and they prefer to accomplish this objective by using strategies tied to their past experiences of themselves and their social world. Change is linked to the person's perceived past, producing continuity in inner psychological characteristics as well as in social behavior and in social circumstances. Continuity is thus a grand adaptive strategy that is promoted by both individual preference and social approval.

"The disengagement theory of aging claims that elderly people systematically disengage from social roles due to the inevitability of death."

Abstract:

Disengagement theory was one of the first theories of aging developed by social scientists. It was originally formulated by Elaine Cumming and Warren Earl Henry in their 1961 book *"Growing Old"*. In *"Growing Old"*, Cumming and Henry develop a logical argument for why older adults would naturally disengage from society. They formulate their argument along nine postulates to explain why it is rational for individuals who know that death is approaching and who have seen friends of their age pass to begin to anticipate their own deaths and disengage. Unfortunately, little empirical data for their claims is provided.

Source: Boundless. "Disengagement Theory." Boundless Sociology. Boundless, 26 May. 2016. Retrieved 20 Jun. 2016 from https://www.boundless.com/sociology/textbooks/boundless-sociology-textbook/aging-18/the-functionalist-perspective-on-aging-128/disengagement-theory-721-9147/

Notes

About the Author

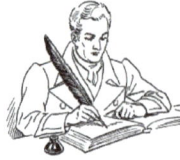

"And death shall have no dominion..."

Over the past 7 years in China, Bromme Hampton Cole has been tagged by Asian journalists as a transformational leader, disruptive businessman and at times, a dissident entrepreneur. He outright rejects such characterizations as superficial. They are, however, a result of his maverick ideas and inextinguishable enthusiasm which has been shaking up China's aged-care health industry in effective ways. Bromme is zealously devoted to challenging the status quo, seeking overlooked opportunities in the healthcare value chain and implementing dynamic solutions. In a recent interview, the Straits Times called him "...the rarest of businessmen: a healthcare iconoclast." Bromme finds this portrayal slightly eccentric, but welcomes its ostensible percipience.

Out of the boardroom, Bromme satisfies his passion for adventure with a keen enthusiasm for custom motorcycles. But when among close friends and staff, Bromme transposes; he is beguiling and reflective, visualizing his role as a force multiplier within the senior healthcare industry. And in quieter moments, he is a voracious scribe; he has written two books on China's massive demographic transition; his third and final in the series is forthcoming. Yet in simplest terms, Bromme is best explained as an intrepid idealist who thrives on the edge of a power curve...never yielding, always progressing and unconcerned with mistakes. He openly acknowledges being mercurial, pensive to the point of absentmindedness and an impenitent aesthete.

He has several businesses in China, among them "iHuHuHu", the revolutionary mobile healthcare APP, "WeBamboo", China's first volunteer platform and "Care Expo", China's most important B2B aged-care conference and trade show.

He can be contacted via Linkedin or brommecole@yahoo.com.

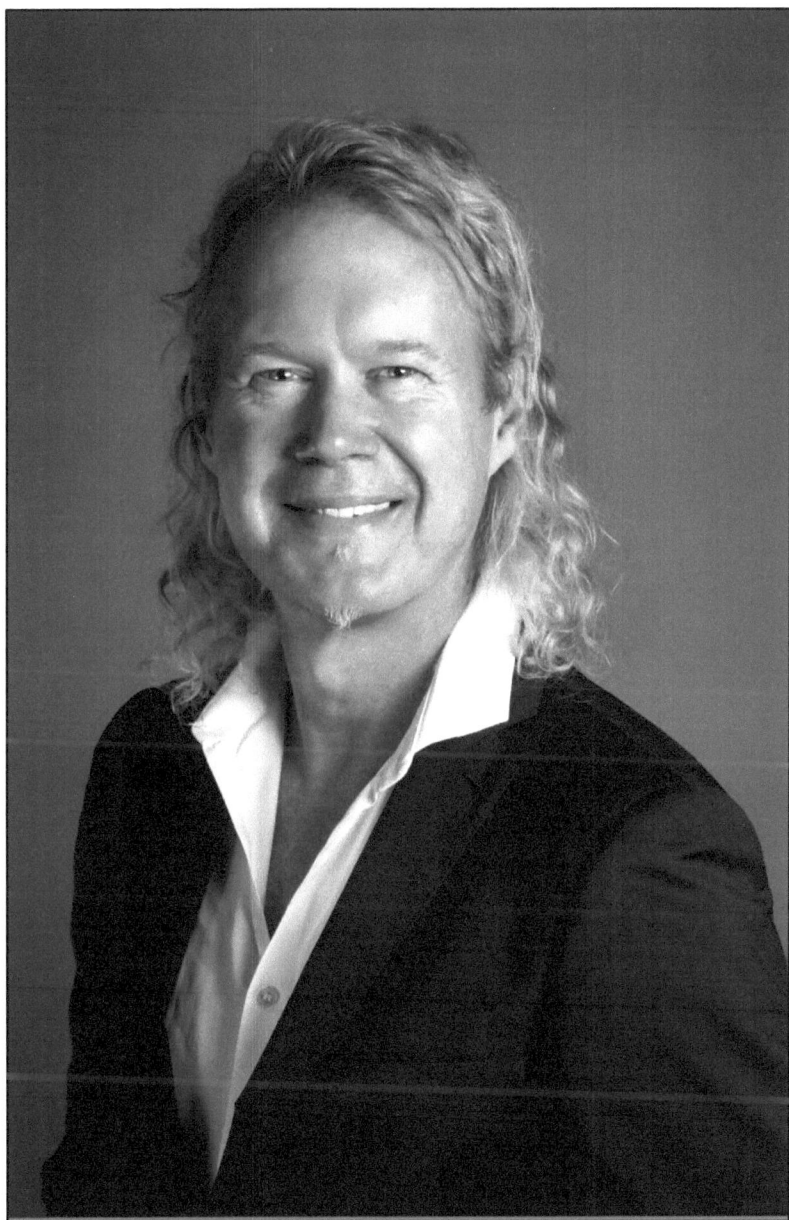

www.ingramcontent.com/pod-product-compliance
Lightning Source LLC
Chambersburg PA
CBHW040124270326
41926CB00001B/10